# After Adoption

Few children nowadays are placed for adoption without any form of contact planned with birth relatives and professional practitioners are increasingly advocating the value of direct rather than indirect contact. Practice has outstripped evidence in this respect and not enough is known about how contact arrangements actually work out, particularly for older children adopted from state care. Such children have often experienced neglect and abuse, and they have frequently been adopted without parental agreement.

Based on research with a large number of adoptive parents, children and birth relatives, *After Adoption* considers the impact of direct (face-to-face) post-adoption contact on all concerned in such cases. It also:

- discusses the development of adoption policy and law, particularly with regard to their legal and social consequences
- reviews the research evidence on adopted children's contact with their birth families
- explores through interviews: participants' feelings about adoption and direct contact; their relationships with each other; what hinders and what helps in maintaining beneficial contact.

*After Adoption* challenges readers to re-think the relationship between adoption and the possibility of direct post-adoption contact and at the same time provides a comprehensive understanding of adoption issues. It is a timely and valuable addition to the literature on adoption, making a substantial contribution to policy and practice.

**Carole Smith and Janette Logan** are both Senior Lecturers in the Department of Applied Social Science at the University of Manchester.

# After Adoption

Direct contact and relationships

**Carole Smith and Janette Logan**

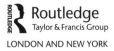

LONDON AND NEW YORK

First published 2004
by Routledge
11 New Fetter Lane, London EC4P 4EE

Simultaneously published in the USA and Canada
by Routledge
29 West 35th Street, New York, NY 10001

*Routledge is an imprint of the Taylor & Francis Group*

© 2004 Carole Smith and Janette Logan

Typeset in Times New Roman by
Keystroke, Jacaranda Lodge, Wolverhampton
Printed and bound in Great Britain by
MPG Books Ltd, Bodmin, Cornwall

*British Library Cataloguing in Publication Data*
A catalogue record for this book is available from the British Library

*Library of Congress Cataloging in Publication Data*
A catalog record for this book has been requested

ISBN 0–415–28221–7 (pbk)
ISBN 0–415–28208–X (hbk)

# Contents

# Illustrations

## Figures

## Tables

# Acknowledgements

We would like to thank the following for their help in completing the research and producing this book: the Nuffield Foundation, which funded our research; all the adoptive parents, children and birth relatives who gave us their time to discuss adoption and contact – we wish them well; Pam Walker, our research assistant for six months, without whose enthusiasm and persistence the work would never have been completed; our secretary, Alison, who rescued us when the chips were down.

Carole would especially like to thank her daughter, Joan, for her patience and tolerance in living with a mother who only occasionally emerged from her study to see if the cobwebs had taken over the house or if anyone had died from starvation.

# 1 Adoption in context
## Social change and openness

### Adoption: the pace and nature of change

Adoption is one of the most fascinating topics to have attracted our attention, first as social-work practitioners and subsequently as researchers and academics. It represents a remarkable relationship between the legal definition and effects of an adoption order and the way in which adopters and their children develop bonds of love and attachment through the everyday social construction of family life. Adoption demonstrates a sense of optimism about society's ability to engineer happy outcomes for children while, at the same time, it deprives birth parents of any legal parental status and historically has rendered them strangers to their children. As Fratter and her colleagues comment, adoption tends to 'arouse strong emotions because of its potentialities for happy or tragic outcomes' (Fratter *et al.* 1991: 13). We are clearly not alone and share our fascination for adoption with numerous commentators to whom we refer during the course of this book. It is apparent that the media and public are also interested in adoption 'stories'. Newspaper coverage of adoption has become so extensive that, in 1999, British Agencies for Adoption and Fostering established a monthly subscription service to distribute press cuttings about adoption and associated topics.

Since its legal inception in 1926 (1930 in Scotland), adoption has acted as a barometer of social change, reflecting and responding to issues of public and political interest. This book is particularly concerned with society's interest in the role of adoption and post-adoption contact between children and their birth families. In 1964 Krugman observed 'the field of adoption seems now to be so characterised by outspokenness, rapid growth and change that one sometimes feels new programmes are in existence before old ones have been evaluated' (p. 268). More recently, Fratter *et al.* (1991: 7) have similarly noted that the 'history of adoption over the past 50 years is truly remarkable' and 'the speed and magnitude of the changes that have occurred are amazing'. The pace has not slowed down since 1991. Since then, the Children Act 1989 has been implemented and in December 1991 the United Kingdom ratified the United Nations Convention on the Rights of the Child. Next, the Interdepartmental Working Group (1992) reported on its review of adoption law. A White Paper on adoption was published in 1993 (Secretary of State for Health 1993), followed by an adoption Bill

(Department of Health and Welsh Office 1996), which failed to reach Parliament when the Conservatives lost the general election in 1997.

Meanwhile, the Department of Health (1996a and 1998a) was directing local authorities to give adoption a more central role in planning for children looked after by the state. In February 1996 the Department contacted directors of social services reminding them about thousands of children who had benefited from adoption and pointing out that 'adoption and adoptive families should be regarded positively as an important child care resource' (1996a: 2). Later that year the Social Services Inspectorate (Department of Health 1996b) published its overview of local authority adoption services. Evidence indicated poor strategic planning for service provision, a failure to conduct three yearly reviews as required, an apparent disregard of adoption as part of mainstream services for looked-after children and avoidable delays in planning permanent placements. This was followed in August 1998 by further guidance where the Department states that an approach, which relentlessly pursues rehabilitation without a clear timetable for making alternative plans, 'lacks proper balance'. In this context adoption should be viewed as 'an important service for children, offering a positive and beneficial outcome' (1998a: 2). By this time the Department was getting tough and guidance was issued under section 7 of the Local Authority and Social Services Act 1970, which requires compliance unless local conditions demonstrate that alternative arrangements are appropriate.

Although the New Labour government initially showed little urgency about expediting adoption law reform, several factors combined to prepare the ground for policy and legislative change. Information entered the public domain showing that looked-after children were significantly disadvantaged in terms of their emotional well-being, educational achievement, opportunities to experience placement stability and secure attachments, and their ability to function as socially and economically competent adults (Secretary of State for Health 1998). The government responded swiftly to concerns about poor outcomes for looked-after children and initiated the Quality Protects programme for England in late 1998 and its equivalent for Wales in 1999. Initially a three- and subsequently a five-year programme, Quality Protects provides additional resources to help local authorities meet the government's national objectives for children's services. The objective of 'ensuring that children are securely attached to carers capable of providing safe and effective care for the duration of childhood' (Secretary of State for Health 1998: 111) is of central importance and clearly relevant to adoption practice. Additionally, it was also becoming evident that children were too frequently abused rather than protected while they were being looked after by the state (Utting 1991 and 1997; Department of Health 1998b).

However, it was the 'Waterhouse Report' (Waterhouse 2000) that finally prompted government action on adoption. This report on institutional abuse in North Wales pointed to the lack of proactive planning and 'drift' as a significant factor in the state's failure to adequately protect children in its care. Once again, adoption moved to centre stage. In February 2000 the Prime Minister announced that he 'would personally lead a thorough review of adoption policy, to ensure we [are] making the best use of adoption as an option to meet the needs of children looked after by local authorities' (Performance and Innovation Unit 2000: 3). Fuel was added to the flames of urgent anticipation when the Social Services Inspectorate (Department of Health 2000) reported on its national survey of local authority adoption services. The survey was supplemented by detailed data collection in thirty-four authorities and inspections of adoption services in ten councils. Results indicated a wide variation in local authorities' use of adoption for looked-after children and in some authorities excessive delays in making adoption plans, placing children with prospective adopters and achieving adoption orders. As the Social Services Inspectorate was collating its findings, these became available to the Performance and Innovation Unit's review of adoption services. The Performance and Innovation Unit reported in July 2000 and made practice and legislative proposals for tackling key barriers to adoption. It concluded that 'the government should promote an increase in adoption for looked-after children, and that there is scope to increase the number of adoptions each year' (Performance and Innovation Unit 2000: 5). A White Paper followed in December 2000 (Secretary of State for Health 2000) and the Adoption and Children Bill was presented to Parliament in March 2001. The general election interrupted progress of the March Bill but the Queen's speech in June 2001 reaffirmed the government's intention to introduce legislation designed to reform adoption law. A second Adoption and Children Bill was introduced in October 2001. Following parliamentary discussion and amendment, the Bill received royal assent in November 2002 to become the Adoption and Children Act 2002. Harris-Short (2001: 407) characterises the government's adoption policy as reflecting a 'child saving rhetoric'. She says:

> The PIU report has a clear, unequivocal message: too many children are in care for too long; these children need a family who can meet their needs on a permanent basis; adoption can provide such a family; adoption law, therefore, needs to be reformed to achieve more adoptions more quickly.

The government appears to have provided ample evidence for this interpretation. For example, in his introduction to the Performance and Innovation Unit's report (2000: 3) the Prime Minister said 'it is hard to overstate the importance of a stable and loving family life for children. That is why I want more children to benefit from adoption'. When the Secretary of State for Health introduced the White Paper on adoption to Parliament in December 2000, he commented on the importance of 'safety, stability and loving care', which could be provided through adoption for looked-after children unable to return to their birth families. He concluded:

> More than 28,000 children have been in care continuously for more than two years . . . These children need a better chance in life. They deserve a better deal. Adoption can provide just such a new start in life for a looked after child. Too often adoption has been seen as a last resort when it should have been considered as a first resort.
>
> (*Hansard*, volume 360, column 579)

To be fair, it had been acknowledged for years that adoption law required reform. Prior to royal assent for the Adoption and Children Act 2002, adoption was governed by the Adoption Act 1976 and the Adoption Agencies Regulations 1983. Practice in adoption had moved on considerably since 1976 and it was argued that adoption legislation should more closely reflect principles in the Children Act 1989 (Ryburn 1992; King 1994; Roll 2001) and the United Nations Convention on the Rights of the Child (Lansdown 1994). Indeed, many proposals in the 1996 Bill introduced by the Conservative government were repeated in the Adoption and Children Bill of October 2001 (Barton 2001) and remain in the 2002 Act. However, throughout the process of policy and legislative reform it is impossible to escape a sense of urgency about making adoption plans for a greater number of looked-after children and implementing plans more quickly. In its White Paper (Secretary of State for Health, 2000: 5) the government promised to invest £66.5 million over three years to improve adoption services. It set a target for a 40 per cent (preferably 50 per cent) increase over 1999 levels in the number of looked-after children adopted by 2005. Since 1974, the number of children adopted from care has remained reasonably stable at around 2,000 each year. This represents about 1.5 per cent of the care population in 1970 and about 4 per cent in 2000. The number of looked-after children who have left care through adoption has gradually increased since the implementation of Quality Protects in 1998 from 2,100 in that year to 3,400 in 2002 (Department of Health 2002a). Comments in the Social Services Performance Assessment Framework Indicators for 2000/1 and 2001/2 (Department of Health 2001a and 2002b) refer approvingly to the trajectory, which puts local authorities on track to surpass the government's 'if possible' target of a 50 per cent increase in children adopted from care. To help matters along and to standardise good practice across local authorities, the National Adoption Standards were published in August 2001 with an implementation date of April 2003 (Department of Health 2001b). The Standards require a plan for permanence to be made at every child's statutory review no later than four months after they become looked after and identify time limits within which stages of the adoption process must be completed. In December 2001 the Secretary of State for Health announced a further public-service agreement target on adoption (LAC(2001)33). By 31 March 2005, at least 95 per cent of looked-after children should be placed for adoption within twelve months of a local authority making the decision that adoption is in their best interests. This represents an increase over the 81 per cent of children for whom this target was achieved in 2001.

Adoption services cannot have experienced such pressure since the peak year of 1968 when nearly 25,000 adoption orders were made (Grey 1971). At that time the vast majority of adoptions were arranged by voluntary societies, which were responsible for placing over 9,000 babies a year (Fratter *et al.* 1991: 8). The annual number of adoptions is now much reduced, beginning with a downward trend from 1969 when 23,700 adoption orders were granted. In 1974, 22,400 children were adopted and between 1991 and 1998 the numbers fell inexorably from 6,901 to 4,617 (Registrar General 2001). The 1993 White Paper on adoption noted adoption's changing role. It pointed out that in 1997 nearly 13,000 children were adopted, of whom 3,000 (23 per cent) were babies under a year old. By 1991, the number of babies adopted had fallen to under 900 (12 per cent) of the total. Additionally, step-parent and relative applications accounted for about half of all adoption orders, indicating a persistent trend. Clearly, adoption has ceased to be primarily a service for unmarried mothers, babies and childless couples. Looked-after children who are adopted had an average age of 5 years, 9 months in 1995 and 4 years, 4 months in 1999 (Performance and Innovation Unit 2000: 12). They are likely to be placed for adoption because of abuse and/or neglect and to have spent well over a year in temporary placement(s) before joining their adoptive families. Many children have 'complex special needs associated with medical problems, severe emotional difficulties, challenging behaviours, sibling group membership and particular racial/ethnic characteristics' (Department of Health 2000: 2). In its survey, which included 1,801 children looked after by 116 local authorities, British Agencies for Adoption and Fostering found that one or both parents contested adoption plans for 71 per cent of children in the sample (Ivaldi 2000: 51).

It is evident that the government has high aspirations for adoption and for the future of children who cease to be looked after through this route to permanence. Between 1950 and 1980 researchers, particularly in Britain, the USA and Sweden, published numerous studies that attempted to identify factors associated with adoption outcome. Although the studies varied methodologically, they reported a high rate of success (around 75 per cent) for placement stability and children's adjustment in their adoptive families. These studies generated an optimistic attitude towards adoption, particularly where they suggested that adopted children suffered fewer developmental problems and lower rates of disrupted placements than their peers who were fostered or placed in residential care. More recently, however, studies indicate that while overall disruption rates are lower for adoption than long-term fostering, age at placement is significantly related to placement stability in both groups. Fratter *et al.* (1991: 53) conclude that 'when age at placement was held constant, there was no significant difference in breakdown rates between adoption or permanent foster placements'. The interpretation of outcome studies is a complicated business and readers who wish to explore this area are referred to Kadushin (1970), Thoburn (1990), Triseliotis *et al.* (1997), Parker (1999) and Triseliotis (2002) for a discussion of relevant literature. Reporting on the Prime Minister's review of adoption, the Performance and Innovation Unit (2000: 16) concluded 'there is no suggestion that adoption outcomes are worse than the alternatives. There is a well established evidence base demonstrating that adopted children do well, if not better, than those in the general population.' One advantage that adopted children do appear to have over their fostered counterparts is a greater sense of security and belonging. This experience derives not only from a distinction in legal status, but from the qualitatively different nature of relationships and mutual expectations within foster and adoptive families (Triseliotis 1983; Hill *et al.* 1989; Bohman and Sigvardson 1990; Triseliotis and Hill 1990).

Despite a vast amount of activity and change since the first Adoption Act was passed in 1926, successive policy and legislative developments have largely failed to tackle the issue of continuing contact between adopted children and their birth families. It has been left to practitioners, researchers and academics to explore the desirability of contact and to articulate the need for policy change to support or require contact arrangements. The current debate about openness and contact may best be understood as it has developed historically. It has gained momentum in response to the changing role of adoption, our understanding of the relationship between contact, identity and children's well-being and evolving expectations about the rights, obligations and responsibilities that parents have towards their children. This chapter will consider these questions. Chapter 2 will go on to discuss available research evidence in relation to openness and contact and Chapter 3 will consider how policy and law have responded to this ongoing debate.

## Adoption practice: openness and secrecy in adoption arrangements

First of all we need to clarify what is involved in references to openness and contact in adoptive and birth-family relationships. Triseliotis (1991: 20) refers to 'open adoption' as involving birth parents in the choice of adoptive parents for their child. Birth-parent involvement may extend to include an initial meeting with prospective adopters. In New Zealand, where these arrangements are well established, initial meetings between birth and prospective adoptive parents enable them to negotiate further opportunities for openness, which may include continuing direct or indirect contact following adoption (Iwanek 1987; Dominick 1988; Rockel and Ryburn 1988). Later, Triseliotis (1993: 48) defines open adoption as follows:

> Open adoption may simply involve the exchange of information and photographs; or constitute an initial meeting between birth and adoptive parent(s); or involve an initial meeting and subsequent exchange of correspondence and photographs; or be of intermittent contact, say once every year or longer; and finally it may include continued contact and a close relationship between the two sets of families.

Later still, Triseliotis *et al.* (1997: 71) refer to open adoption as an umbrella term that includes arrangements 'from the most minimal sharing of information to continued visits between birth and adoptive families'. So, open adoption is usually understood to include the possibility of ongoing contact in some form. However, it should be remembered that contact is not equivalent to 'access' and may involve indirect contact where one- or two-way information is mediated by a third party, usually the adoption agency. Similarly, direct (face-to-face) contact may be controlled insofar as arrangements are made by the agency, meetings are held in a 'contact centre' or some other neutral venue and families do not exchange addresses or telephone numbers. These differences bear on a complementary interpretation of openness, which emphasises adoptive parents' attitudes rather than the accomplishment of practical arrangements. In this situation, adoptive parents are comfortable with adoption, understand the importance of birth-family links and are keen to consider how best to maintain a sense of continuity for their adopted children. Thus, an apparently open adoption with direct contact may be attitudinally closed if adopters feel resentful, threatened and unwilling to incorporate a child's pre-adoption experiences and relationships into their family life. Semi-open adoption is described by Triseliotis (1991: 20) as involving the provision of full, but non-identifying information, about their respective families to birth and prospective adoptive parents. These arrangements do not extend to meetings between families (Fish and Speirs 1990). In any event, open adoption is distinct from closed adoption where there is no contact at all. Agencies pass only minimal information about adopters to birth parents and adopters are given little information about birth families and their child's history. Open adoption is not a new phenomenon in some cultures where adoption arrangements were publicly acknowledged and both sets of parents were well known to each other. For example Baran *et al.* (1976: 98) refer to practice in Hawaii:

> The child, in essence, belonged to two families openly and proudly: the family that gave him his birthright and the family that nurtured and protected him. Many well known Hawaiians have been raised in the Landi system and they speak openly of their dual identity. Their loyalty appears to be with their adoptive families, but they also take great pride in the connection with their birth families.

Similarly, Rockel and Ryburn (1988) describe the Maori system where adoptions were public knowledge and children's relationships with their birth parents were well known and understood. History suggests that, as law has increasingly come to govern adoption arrangements, cultural variations on openness have been superseded by a legally imposed uniformity in which secrecy has played a central role.

Many commentators agree that for several decades following the 1926 Adoption Act in England and Wales, legislation and practice effectively drew a veil of secrecy over adoption. This approach was designed to ensure adoptive families' security against any subsequent interference from birth parents and an escape from the shame of illegitimacy for birth mothers and their children (Haimes and Timms 1985: 2; Fratter *et al.* 1991: 7; Triseliotis 1991: 19; Ivaldi 2000: 1). The Registrar General was directed to maintain a separate register in which details of adoption orders were recorded in such a way that entries could be cross-referenced with the register of births. Until implementation of section 26 of the Children Act 1975, access to information from an adopted child's original birth entry was only possible through obtaining a court order on the basis of exceptional circumstances. In Scotland, however, the first Adoption Act of 1930 allowed adopted people, of at least 17 years old, to identify the connection between entries relating to their adoption order and to their birth registration. Armed with information about their birth registration, they were able to apply to the Registrar General for a copy of their original birth certificate.

While observations about secrecy may be generally accurate, it was not until well after 1926 that all the loopholes were closed. For example, birth parents had a right to know the identity of adopters until a private member's bill in 1949 successfully introduced the serial number procedure into court rules, thus ensuring anonymity for adoption applicants (Triseliotis, 1970: 2; Ryburn, 1997a: 31). Adoption placements with non-relatives through a third party or directly between parents and prospective adopters were not prohibited until the Children Act 1975 and the consolidating Adoption Act of 1976. A survey of 3,400 adoption applications in 1966 (Grey 1971) identified 13,330 (82 per cent) agency placements, 1,035 (6 per cent) placements arranged by a third party and 1,740 (11 per cent) placements arranged directly between birth and prospective adoptive parents (excluding parental applications). Although a proportion of these 'independent' placements were made with relatives, birth parents and adopters were able to meet quite naturally or to exchange information through a third party – and this was years before agencies began to advocate open adoption. Rockel and Ryburn (1988) also note that the first adoption legislation in New Zealand, passed in 1881, aimed only to provide a legal foundation for adoption. It was only subsequent policy, culminating in the 1955 Adoption Act, which increasingly limited access to information and established secrecy between parties to adoption arrangements. Avery (1998) identifies comparable developments in the USA where early state legislation was not concerned with issues relating to confidentiality in adoption.

## The changing role of adoption: difference, identity and 'telling'

Early adoption practice paid scant attention to what later became acknowledged as complex issues for birth parents and adoptive families. The 1926 Adoption Act was designed to establish legal recognition of adoption and made no provision for regulating the activities of voluntary societies, which increasingly arranged adoptions. It was assumed that the motivation to adopt was sufficient to ensure conscientious parenting. The first committee to consider the need for adoption legislation (Hopkinson Committee 1921) said that the desire to bring up a child 'is one of the strongest feelings of human nature and is in itself the best guarantee for the welfare of the adopted child'. The Horsburgh Committee (1937) was set up to investigate concerns about poor practice and found it necessary to recommend that adoption societies should concentrate on the personal suitability of adopters as well as their material circumstances. Early literature is replete with enthusiastic references to baby placements and sympathetic comments about the plight of childless couples. Ellison (1958: 65) expresses something of these attitudes when she remarks 'every sort of baby is asked for – chubby, tiny, curly haired, lively, blue eyed. Even one with a squint is sometimes wanted'. Bowerbank (1970: 35) notes that case papers recording adoption societies' work during and after the Second World War: 'Suggest that almost any adopter furnishing satisfactory references was acceptable and interviews were mainly concerned with the sex, colouring and suitability of babies . . . Letters from the society were full of warm thanks to applicants for offering homes to babies.' In the USA there was a similar assumption that people who chose to parent a child through adoption were likely to be 'of more than ordinary emotional depth, greater than common seriousness in their relation to life and to each other, more than usual conscientiousness' (Lockridge 1947: 32). Witmer *et al.* (1963: 47) describe how the introduction of greater regulation in the USA was 'bitterly fought' in some quarters, particularly in relation to an increasing emphasis on the investigation and supervision of prospective adopters. Adopters could escape investigation and surveillance if they opted to accept children without an agency's help. However, they were urged to use adoption agencies to ensure the health and sound background of their babies and to facilitate matching (Lockridge 1947; Ellison 1958; Kirk 1964; Tizard 1977).

For many years openness in adoption was simply not an issue that crossed anyone's mind. Insofar as there was any concern about a child's sense of identity, this was resolved by advising adopters to tell children about their legal status. This matter tended, however, to be left to adoptive parents' good sense. The Hurst Committee (1954) was established in 1953 to review adoption law. It recommended that applications to adopt should be accompanied by an undertaking to tell the child about his or her adoption. Subsequent legislation (Adoption Act 1958) failed to incorporate this proposal but arrangements were made to provide all adopters with an explanatory memorandum. The memorandum remarked 'you may prefer not to tell him anything; but that would be unwise, because he would be likely to find out himself sooner or later and if you had not told him, the discovery might be a shock' (Home Office 1959). Haimes and Timms (1985) note that the memorandum failed to acknowledge the complexities relating to the process of 'telling' or the significance of this information for children. Advice to practitioners about helping adoptive parents with 'telling' had achieved greater sophistication by 1970 (Advisory Council on Child Care 1970). It recommended that adopters should be given education and support to manage 'telling' sensitively and appropriately and pointed out that discussing adoption with children constitutes an ongoing activity rather than a one-off admission. Additionally, it was important to record a 'social history' from birth parent(s) to satisfy children's ongoing requests for information. The Advisory Council on Child Care (1970: 22) very tentatively suggested that a limited degree of (indirect) contact between birth parents and adopters might be helpful.

David Kirk (1964) was influential in generating an awareness that adoption might be rather more complicated than placing babies with well-meaning citizens and leaving them to get on with it. He argued that adoptive parents must confront several dilemmas. First, he identified 'enchantment versus disenchantment'. Adopters must decide how far to acknowledge to themselves and others that they have a particular legal and social status distinguishing them from birth parents. Second, 'integration versus differentiation' requires adopters to consider how far they will acknowledge their child's adoptive status by incorporating reminders about adoption into their everyday lives. Third, 'ignorance versus knowledge about the child's background' asks whether adopters will forget or bury pre-adoption information about their child. Fourth, 'reproductive morals versus the principle of respect for individual personality' concerns explaining why the child was adopted without conveying negative judgements about birth parents. Patterns of managing these dilemmas were characterised as 'acknowledgement of difference' and 'rejection of difference'. Kirk suggested it was important to help adopters develop a willingness and ability to acknowledge the difference between adoptive and birth parenthood. This would facilitate communication about adoption, comfort with the child's adoptive status, a sense of openness and, ultimately, contribute to successful outcomes. Importantly, Kirk emphasised that prospective adopters required education, preparation and support for undertaking the role of adoptive parenthood. Group-work was a useful medium for achieving understanding and changing attitudes. This represents an entirely different approach to early selection methods based on minimal investigation and to later attempts at assessing whether applicants had the 'right' attitudes, history and family circumstances to make competent parents. In 1967 David and Ruth Kirk visited Britain to disseminate their ideas and, according to Rowe and Lambert (1973: 112), they 'had a profound influence on the thinking of adoption workers'.

Clinicians and theorists began to develop an interest in the psychodynamic basis of adoptive relationships in which factors affecting the child's sense of identity and emotional health became issues of central concern. They discussed at length the implications of Freud's (1957) 'family romance' theory for the appropriate timing of revelations about adoption and the child's ability to identify with adoptive parents. Discussions centred on circumstances that might prompt children to split an awareness of their parents as good and bad, permissive and restrictive, giving and withholding and to attribute 'good' characteristics to one set of parents and 'bad' characteristics to the other. There is an enormous literature on this topic which is illustrated by Peller (1961), Lawton and Gross (1964), Schwartz (1970), Sorosky *et al.* (1975) and Wieder (1977). Anticipating these issues, Clothier (1943: 222) suggested that an adopted child without links to their birth family had 'lost the thread of family continuity'. Loss of the biological mother 'appears as an unknown void, separating the adopted child from his fellows whose blood ties them to the past as well as to the future'. Later, Sants's (1964) influential work developed this theme. He defined the 'genealogically bewildered' child as having no or only uncertain knowledge about his or her biological parents. Sants argued that this dislocation of experience and knowledge hampers the growing child's ability to place themselves in relation to their biological heritage and the absence of a genetic link with their adoptive parents may impede appropriate identification. There was thus a growing debate among academics, researchers and clinicians about the nature and significance of identity issues for adopted children. This promoted a recognition that telling children about their adoptive status required sensitivity, continuity of discussion and attention to 'timing' in terms of the child's maturity and degree of understanding (Brodzinsky 1984). 'Telling' was clearly not as straightforward as had once been assumed! These developments prompted much discussion about how far and in what ways adoptive parenthood was distinct from, and more problematic than birth parenthood (Rowe 1966; Kellmer Pringle 1967; Jaffee and Fanshel 1970; Reeves and Dolan 1978).

Two further developments had a profound impact on the role of adoption. These necessarily influenced practitioners' understanding of adoptive parenthood and their expectation that adopters should acknowledge children's links with their birth families. First, as the number of 'baby adoptions' was falling, attention became focused on children drifting in care. Parker (1971) argued that social workers collectively were failing to plan adequately for such children. In 1973 Rowe and Lambert published their blockbuster *Children Who Wait*. Their sample of thirty-three statutory and voluntary agencies and 2,812 children in care yielded 626 (22 per cent) children who were waiting for permanent family placements – 7,000 children on a national basis. These children had 'special needs'. Two-thirds were over school age, a quarter were black, they frequently had behaviour problems and/or developmental delay, and many needed families willing to accept their siblings. Even more alarming, however, Rowe and Lambert found that 61 per cent of the children in their study were expected to grow up in care. As Rowe and Lambert were reporting on their research, information from the USA indicated that practitioners there were attacking this problem from two related directions. Agencies were initiating decisive permanency planning involving working with parents through contracts, time-limited goals and intensive support to effect rehabilitation. However, lack of progress towards rehabilitation resulted in early decisions about alternative plans in which adoption played a significant role. Around this time Goldstein *et al.* (1973 and 1980) added fuel to the fire by suggesting that placements should be secured through adoption once a child's caretaker had effectively become their psychological parent and ties to birth parents had lost their significance for the child. What was known as the 'permanency move-ment' took off in Britain in the late 1970s and extended into the 1980s (McKay 1980; Hussell and Monaghan 1982; Morris 1984). Together with planning for permanence, practitioners in the USA were also recruiting families for children previously considered difficult or impossible to place. The American agency, Spaulding for Children, is generally credited with beginning this pioneering work and its Director Kay Donley came to Britain to encourage similar practice here. Phillida Sawbridge visited Spaulding for Children in 1972 and began to promote its approach in the UK (Association of British Adoption Agencies 1975). Adoption became possible for a greater number of children and these included children who might otherwise have been left to grow up in care (Churchill *et al.* 1979; Sawbridge 1983; Macaskill 1985). Debates about 'acknowledgement of difference' and children's links with their birth families became of acute significance as more adopters accepted older children and others with special needs. Trans-racial placements raised questions about the ability of white families to give children a thorough sense of their black identity, pride in their heritage and skills to deal with endemic racism. Older children had established relationships with their birth families and abuse or neglect could not eradicate memories and important attachments.

One of the most significant changes in adoption practice over the years must be the transition from thinking that 'telling' was a sufficient response to children's loss of their birth families to an approach that calls for open adoption and con-tinuing contact. Some commentators suggested relatively early on that continuing contact might be in the best interests of a limited number of children (Haimes and

Timms, 1985; Triseliotis 1985). However, since 1990 post-adoption contact has become a central issue for practitioners, academics and researchers. It is far from constituting an unproblematic feature of adoption practice and the debate continues about what kind of contact, for which children, under what circumstances and with whom it should be arranged.

## Identity issues in context

It is interesting that concern about identity, genealogical connectedness and the role of continuing contact are being expressed across different situations that involve children's separation from parents or a lack of knowledge about their genetic inheritance. Courts have been struggling with how best to resolve disputes about contact between divorcing and separating parents and case law has now developed principles to guide judgments in these situations (Advisory Board on Family Law 2001 and 2002). In the Court of Appeal Sir Thomas Bingham said 'where parents of a child are separated and the child is in the day to day care of one of them, it is almost always in the interests of the child that he or she should have contact with the other parent' (*Re O (A Minor) (Contact: Imposition of Conditions)* [1995] 2 FLR 124). This principle is mediated by a court's duty to treat the child's welfare as paramount and by any 'cogent reasons' why contact may not be in a child's best interests. Similarly, there is an ongoing debate about the rights of children born as the result of donor insemination to have information about their genetic fathers. In 1984 the Warnock Committee acknowledged that secrecy could 'undermine the whole network of family relationships' and indicated it was 'wrong to deceive children about their origins' (Department of Health and Social Security 1984: 21). Children born after the introduction of the Human Fertilisation and Embryology Act 1990 have a right of access, when they reach eighteen, to basic non-identifying information about their genetic fathers held by the Human Fertilisation and Embryology Authority. Some countries, for example Sweden, Austria and Victoria (Australia), have introduced legislation allowing 'donor offspring' a right of access to identifying information about donors in cases of assisted conception. However, there is still much discussion about the relative rights of donors to anonymity and of children born through donor-assisted conception to information. In December 2001 the government launched a public consultation about what information, if any, should be available to 'donor off- spring' born since the Human Fertilisation and Embryology Act was implemented in August 1991 (Department of Health 2001c). Many aspects of this debate echo early issues in adoption relating to secrecy, telling, privacy and children's needs for genealogical continuity and information (Blyth, 1999).

While we cannot explore this in detail here, it is tempting to speculate about why identity issues have come to attract such professional and public interest. Identity is a complicated concept. It refers to the construction of a sense of self and personal uniqueness through awareness of particular physical and psychological charac- teristics that both differentiate individuals from each other and link them together. Achievement of identity requires knowledge about social and genetic antecedents and the ability to incorporate personal history into a continuing narrative as self-awareness is mediated through new experiences, relationships and social contexts (Schechter and Bertocci 1990; Brodzinsky *et al.* 1992). Clearly, new developments such as donor-assisted conception throw up equally novel moral and social issues. However, some sociologists explain our concern about identity as a response to broader social changes involving an enormous acceleration in the pace and global scope of change and in the growing complexity of institutional relationships. Individuals have to accomplish a sense of continuity and meaning without access to sources of external reference, like tradition, locality, kinship, community and ritual passage, which were previously available to them (Giddens 1990 and 1991). Similarly, Bauman (1993) and Young (1999) point to the pervasive effects of fragmentation where the self must respond to an increasingly complex network of roles, expert systems proliferate and technology prioritises the means (the 'technological fix') over the ends of its operations. It is argued that these developments generate a self-referential attitude that encourages individualism and a concern with personal identity. This internal reflection seeks to locate the self with reference to a personal biography because external social referents no longer have the capacity to make a significant contribution to our sense of identity. Whatever sociologists may have to suggest, policy-makers, legislators and practitioners must determine a response to the expressed needs of those who experience dislocated relationships and 'genealogical bewilderment'.

## The current debate: openness, contact and adoption

The debate about adoption and continuing contact focuses on three related areas: the child's need for information and continuing knowledge about his or her birth family; the child's right to such information; and the way in which adoption acts to attenuate these opportunities for children. The issues are, however, hotly contested. McWhinnie (1994: 7) suggests about evidence to the Interdepartmental Review of Adoption Law (Interdepartmental Working Group 1992):

> Adoption was not being presented as a positive institution in child care provision, but one that was outmoded and in need of radical overhaul. The arguments put forward for that view are that it does harm to children's sense of identity and that it is a form of injustice perpetrated on birth mothers . . . The idea of 'open adoption' was seen as a solution. It was not, however, debated. It has become a kind of ideology against which no arguments are permissible. I have found no research evidence as to its genuine long-term advisability and certainly none as to its outcome.

Developing this theme, Hughes (1995) argues that there is an unfounded but nevertheless growing professional assumption that direct post-adoption contact is beneficial for children. Taking this view, good practice demands that direct contact should be the preferred option along a continuum of arrangements for enhancing openness. Ryburn (1994: 199) has no doubt that continuing contact is vital for children's well-being. He asserts 'we know unequivocally that the balance of evidence points to the importance of the maintenance of links and contact for those who are adopted, with their original families'. Continuing contact is so important in Ryburn's view that he thinks either the courts should take steps to *enforce* contact after adoption or children should be placed under alternative arrangements (Ryburn 1994, 1997a and 1997b). These might include permanent fostering or a residence order under section 8 of the Children Act 1989. Similarly, he argues that children should be placed with relatives rather than strangers if the latter are unwilling to facilitate birth family contact.

Ryburn and others whose work supports continuing contact (see Fratter *et al.* 1991; chapters in Mullender 1991; Adcock *et al.* 1993; Fratter 1996; Hill and Shaw 1998, Section 111) tend to focus on meeting the child's need for information and ongoing links with their birth families. That is, they suggest contact contributes to children's well-being and their ability to develop a well-balanced sense of identity. Coming from a rather different direction, Lansdown (1994) argues that children have specific rights conferred by the 1989 United Nations Convention on the Rights of the Child. Articles 7, 8, 9 and 12 are of particular relevance to this discussion. Article 7 identifies the child's 'right from birth to a name, the right to acquire a nationality and, as far as possible, the right to know and be cared for by his or her parents'. Article 8 requires States Parties to 'respect the right of the child to preserve his or her identity, including nationality, name and family relations as recognised by law without unlawful interference'. In Article 9 (3) there is a presumption that children separated from their parents have a right to 'maintain personal relations and direct contact with both parents on a regular basis, except if this is contrary to the child's best interests'. Collectively, these Convention rights require policy-makers and practitioners to think carefully about contact arrangements for children who are separated from their parents. Article 12 of the Convention is perhaps the best known for its insistence on children's rights to express their views and, in accordance with their age and maturity, to have them given due weight. It is argued that professionals often make decisions about contact without giving serious consideration to children's wishes and feelings. Lansdown (1994: 70) queries whether total severance resulting from adoption can be consistent with children's Convention rights to an identity, to know their parents and to maintain contact with their birth family. If, however, adoption remains the best option for a child 'the presumption should always be that, as far as is possible, there should be continued and extensive contact with members of the birth family'.

The United Nations Convention on the Rights of the Child has now been sup-plemented by the Human Rights Act 1998, which incorporates the Convention for the Protection of Human Rights and Fundamental Freedoms (commonly known as the European Convention on Human Rights) into domestic law. Adults and children may use the Act to enforce Convention rights against the state in domestic courts, rather than having to appeal to the European Court of Human Rights. Article 8(1) of the Convention states that 'everyone has the right to respect for his private and family life, his home and his correspondence'. This right can only legitimately be violated under conditions set out in Article 8(2). Decisions about the permanent separation of children from their birth families, placement for adoption and arrangements for contact clearly have the potential to violate Article 8(1). To avoid unlawful interference with parents' and children's Article 8(1) rights in the context of adoption and contact, the state must show it has acted in accordance with the law and that its action is necessary in a democratic society for the protection of children's health or morals. Justifying 'necessary' intervention requires the state to explain the grounds for its decision, to show that it has acted fairly and to demonstrate that its action is proportionate to the end it wishes to achieve. Thus, a birth relative or child might complain that a local authority's refusal to make contact arrangements before or after adoption constitutes a *disproportionate* interference with their Article 8(1) rights since a child's need for adoption does not necessarily exclude continuing contact. Although case law is underdeveloped in this area and European jurisprudence has largely privileged parents' rights, the implementation of the Human Rights Act must come to inform decisions about adoption and contact in line with Article 8(1) and (2) (Swindells *et al.* 1999).

It is also argued that the legal effects of an adoption order militate against a proactive attitude to arranging post-adoption contact. An adoption order vests parental responsibility relating to the child in the adopters and extinguishes it in the child's birth parent(s). However, those who wish to promote greater openness in adoption focus their attention on what has been termed the 'legal fiction' expressed in section 39 of the 1976 Adoption Act:

(1) An adopted child shall be treated in law –
　　(a) where the adopters are a married couple, as if he had been born as a child of the marriage (whether or not he was in fact born after the marriage was solemnised);
　　(b) in any other case, as if he had been born to the adopter in wedlock (but not as a child of any actual marriage of the adopter).
(2) An adopted child shall, subject to subsection (3), be treated in law as if he were not the child of any person other than the adopters or adopter.

Section 39 refers only to the legal effects of adoption and was designed to ensure that children could inherit from their adoptive parents under intestacy rules. The 1976 Adoption Act will be superseded by the Adoption and Children Act 2002, section 67 of which conveys essentially the same meaning as section 39 in the former Act. Although the legal status conferred by adoption thus remains similarly expressed, the Explanatory Notes to the 2002 Act point out that section 67 provisions 'do not touch on the biological or emotional ties of an adopted child, nor are they intended to' (paragraph 193). Critics, however, identify the wording of section 39 in the 1976 Act and section 67 in the 2002 Act as supporting a construction of adoption that denies the ongoing significance of birth family members in children's lives. Legislation perpetuates the fiction that adopted children have no other family than their adoptive family (Ryburn 1997a: 29 and 1997b: 29; Lowe 1997: 375). In its review of adoption law, the Law Commission of New Zealand (2000: 43–44) comments specifically on this point. It suggests that current legislation, deeming an adopted child to have been born to adoptive parents, 'is a repugnant and an unnecessary distortion of reality'. The Law Commission recommends that the 'legal fiction' incorporated in section 16 of the 1955 Adoption Act (New Zealand) should be removed from future legislation and that adoption should be defined only in terms of the legal transfer of parental responsibility from birth to adoptive parents. It says:

> This formulation recognises that parental responsibility is being transferred both in law and in fact from the birth parents to the adoptive parents, that a new legal family is being created, *and that a birth family still exists and may have a role in the child's life.*

> (Emphasis added)

Lowe (1997: 383) develops this approach to the role of adoption, particularly for older children. He argues that adoption should be understood as a 'contract' between the birth family, the child and the adoptive parents in which there is an accepted 'pattern of reciprocal obligations between the parties'. Furthermore, adopters should not expect that adoption heralds an end to contact with their child's birth family. Adoptive relationships based on 'reciprocal obligations', with adoption agencies in a supporting role, are likely to require adopters to accept that they 'may not be in complete control of the child's upbringing'. Bridge (1993: 102) also contends that implementing beneficial post-adoption contact necessitates an acknowledgement that children are not exclusively 'owned' *either* by their birth parents *or* subsequently by their adoptive parents. Children may need the legal security of adoption that also incorporates continuity with their social and emotional past. Bridge comments that social attitudes must move away from understanding the status of children as possessions and learn to think about them as being their own persons. The adversarial nature of contested adoptions is also charged with diminishing parties' willingness and ability to negotiate post-adoption contact (Ryburn 1994: 200).

## Conclusion: the debate about contact and new challenges

We have covered a lot of ground in this chapter, ranging over changes in adoption policy and practice, the role of adoption and a developing recognition that identity is an issue for children who are separated from their birth parent(s) or dislocated, in some way, from their genetic background. During this discussion we have also canvassed arguments, which collectively demand a reappraisal of the way in which we understand the legal, social and emotional effects of adoption for birth families, adopters and adopted children. However, as we have pointed out, the debate about post-adoption contact, and particularly direct contact, has not been unequivocally resolved. Contested views about contact are similarly evident in the USA. Grotevant and McRoy (1998: 1) comment that arguments about openness in adoption have 'polarised the adoption community' and led to an 'adversarial relationship between advocates and critics of openness'. It might be reasonably supposed that empirical research would indicate how far post-adoption contact of different kinds is beneficial for children and thus bring the weight of evidence down on one side of the debate. Unfortunately, this supposition is not straightforward and there is further argument about the methodological reliability of studies and interpretation of their findings. We anticipate that our own research will contribute to an understanding of how direct contact impacts on adopters, children and birth relatives and the conditions under which it is experienced as beneficial by those most closely involved. Chapter 2 will clarify what we know, what we think we know and what we do not yet know about post-adoption contact by examining relevant research and considering arguments about its evidential usefulness in supporting contact arrangements.

## Summary

- Adoption was legalised in England and Wales in 1926 and 1930 in Scotland, when it essentially provided a response to the needs of unmarried mothers and involuntarily childless adopters.
- Early adoption practice supported secrecy in adoption arrangements and concentrated only on telling children about their adoptive status. However, a number of factors contributed to the changing role of adoption as the annual number of orders began to decline from 1969. In the late 1970s and early 1980s the 'permanency movement' was imported from the USA and agencies began to place older and other 'special needs' children for adoption. These developments encouraged a professional concern about openness and contact in adoption arrangements.
- Commentators have argued that Articles in the United Nations Convention on the Rights of the Child and the European Convention on Human Rights require recognition of children's rights to information about their birth families and continuing contact with them in the event of separation. It has been argued that the wording of legislation, with reference to the status conferred by adoption, acts to deny the emotional and social significance of birth family members.
- The 'Waterhouse Report' published in 2000 prompted the government to consider adoption policy and the need for legislative reform. Matters moved swiftly with the Prime Minister's review of adoption conducted by the Policy and Innovation Unit, a White Paper on adoption in December 2000, adoption Bills in March and October 2001 and royal assent to the Adoption and Children Act in November 2002.
- Issues associated with openness and post-adoption contact remain contentious. References to openness and contact are definitionally problematic and, while some argue that post-adoption contact is vital for children's well-being and sense of identity, others suggest that little is known about its long-term effects.

# 2 Openness in adoption
## Essential for children's well-being?

### The practice of open adoption and arrangements for contact

In Chapter 1 we referred to growing pressure for policy and practice to recognise the benefits of open adoption and particularly the advantages that are arguably associated with direct contact between children and their birth families. Those who advocate more extensive contact arrangements suggest that the social and legal effects of adoption require a different interpretation to accommodate a continuing role for birth families. Similarly, they argue that social attitudes and professional practice should encourage adoptive parents to relinquish the expectation that adoption consigns a child's birth family to history. Although we do not know how many adoptive families agree to and maintain ongoing contact, it is evident that contact is becoming an increasingly common feature of adoption. Thirty agencies in the north of England reported on post-adoption contact arrangements for 371 children who had been placed for adoption between April 1993 and March 1994 (Department of Health 1995). Direct contact with birth-family members was ongoing for 52 (14 per cent) children, indirect contact for 155 (41 per cent), both direct and indirect contact for 49 (13 per cent) and there was no contact for 115 (31 per cent) children. Thirty-three agencies responded to a request for information about their activities in supporting post-adoption contact. They identified 825 cases where they were facilitating indirect contact for 74 per cent and both direct and indirect contact for 26 per cent of the children. Additionally, agencies were asked to estimate the number of children for whom contact was continuing without their help. Twenty agencies able to answer this question referred to 624 children having post-adoption contact, 222 (36 per cent) of whom were doing so without any agency involvement. The Department of Health (1995: 7) concludes 'there seems little doubt that a more open approach to adoption has been rapidly absorbed into agency practice' although the lack of written policy and procedure suggests that practice had outstripped formal guidance in this respect.

Lowe and colleagues (1999) analysed 226 questionnaires completed by families from forty-one adoption agencies. Families were included in the study where children of 5 years and over had been placed with them for adoption between January 1992 and December 1994. Of these families, 174 (77 per cent) had some form of ongoing contact with birth relatives and for 116 of them the adoption order had already been granted. In eighty-nine (39 per cent) families there was direct ongoing contact with at least one birth relative. In 1993 Ryburn (1996) studied post-adoption contact arrangements for seventy-six children, identified through Parent to Parent Information on Adoption Services, whose adoptions had been contested by their birth parent(s). He was surprised to find a relatively high level of contact following contested adoption proceedings. In thirty-one (42 per cent) cases, children had some form of continuing contact with birth parents and frequently with other relatives. Of these, ten children were in direct contact with one or both birth parents. The adoptive parents of seventeen children indicated that they did not want any contact while the same number were unsure or actively wanted to initiate contact with birth families. Although Murch *et al.* (1993) found fewer cases involving post-adoption contact, their data were extracted from court records. Unless courts had made an order for contact it is unlikely that informal arrangements would have been recorded. Evidence to the Review of Adoption Law (France 1990) suggests a growing international trend towards greater openness in adoption, particularly in New Zealand, the USA, Australia and Canada. Examples of openness noted by France include indirect and direct contact arrangements. She notes that 'some form of ongoing contact between the birth family and the adoptive family is the norm in New Zealand' (1990: 41). Writing in 1993, Etter comments about the USA that 'open adoption, with contact between biological and adoptive parents, has become so common that some suggest it may soon become standard practice' (p. 257). Literature and research clearly indicates that openness has increasingly come to characterise adoption arrangements. However, in the general scheme of openness it is also evident that indirect contact is more frequently preferred to direct (face-to-face) contact (Murch *et al.* 1993; Lowe *et al.* 1999; Neil 2002a).

Advocates of ongoing contact want to see it incorporated into more adoptions and they support an extension of *direct* contact for more children. Howe and Feast (2000: 10) observe 'the recognition that openness in adoption has a range of developmental benefits has led to an increasing number of placements being planned with provision for some form of contact between children and their birth families'. Ryburn suggests that direct contact provides greater benefits for children. He is prepared to extend practice on the basis that 'the research studies suggest that with indirect contact children's information needs begin to be met, but that with direct contact their questions are more likely to be met at a level that is satisfying' (Ryburn 1998: 60). And herein lies the bone of contention. While Ryburn is not alone in believing we have sufficient evidence to assert that contact contributes to children's well-being, others disagree. Ryburn (1998, 1999) and Quinton *et al.* (1998, 1999) have been engaged in an ongoing dispute about what conclusions can legitimately be drawn from relevant research. Quinton *et al.* (1997) considered studies of contact with birth parents where contact was either direct or unspecified in research publications. Their research review was particularly concerned with methodological issues, which necessarily influence the reliability and validity of research data and the degree of confidence that can be attributed to research findings. Quinton *et al.* (1997) suggest that methodologies employed in most studies of post-adoption contact are not sufficiently sophisticated to demonstrate a relationship between different types of contact and long-term benefits for birth relatives, adoptive parents or children. In opposition to Ryburn's position, they conclude:

> In our present state of knowledge it is seriously misleading to think that what we know about contact is at a level of sophistication to allow us to make confident assertions about the benefits to be gained from it, regardless of family circumstances and relationships. At least in the case of permanent placements, the social experiment that is currently underway needs to be recognised as an experiment, not as an example of evidence-based practice.
>
> (Quinton *et al*. 1997: 411)

So, on the one hand we seem to have practice increasingly geared towards arranging indirect and direct contact following adoption and, on the other, we are confronted by uncertainty about whether contact is demonstrably in children's best interests. As we noted in Chapter 1, the evidence does not yet fall clearly on one side of the debate. The remainder of this chapter will consider research findings that are currently available to inform our understanding about the relationship between continuing contact and the well-being of birth relatives, adopters and children.

## Adoption and identity: the need for information and contact

There are now a number of studies that investigate the circumstances under which adopted adults search for information about their backgrounds and/or seek to effect a reunion with their birth families. Researchers have been interested in identifying factors that differentiate between adopted adults who search and those who do not and between those who want information only and those who wish to contact birth parents and other relatives. Information about the relationship between self-esteem, openness in adoption, adoptive family relationships, age at placement and searching behaviour is inconsistent. Research does not provide a clear picture about factors associated with a desire for information or reunion and the characteristics of people who choose not to tread this path (for a review of the literature, see Howe and Feast 2000: 12–24; Roche and Perlesz 2000: 9–10). Additionally, while researchers have been able to study adopted adults who search, it is far more difficult to identify those who do not and thus to make comparisons between the two groups. A further problem is that such research depends on questioning adults who were adopted many years ago when adoption had quite different connotations and attitudes to openness were limited to telling children about their adoptive status (McWhinnie 1967; Triseliotis 1973).

Bearing these difficulties in mind, studies on searching do nonetheless have something to tell us about the needs of adopted children as these are expressed through the retrospective accounts of adopted adults. First, it is evident that women are far more likely to actively seek information and contact with birth families than are men (Stevenson 1976; Gonyo and Watson 1988; Pacheco and Eme 1993; Howe and Feast 2000). Second, high numbers of adults who were adopted around twenty to fifty years ago report that they received relatively little information from their adoptive parents about the circumstances of their adoption or about their birth-family background. They generally felt unable to initiate questions or discussion so that if their adopted parents chose not to raise the subject of adoption, as appeared to be common, children grew up with significant gaps in their knowledge. Third, it is not surprising, therefore, that research frequently identifies similar reasons to explain adopted adults' search for further information. These explanations bear on the need to compete a sense of identity and genealogical continuity. Adopted adults report curiosity about their birth-family origins and the need for information about what constitutes their identity in terms of their physical, psychological and dispositional characteristics (McWhinnie 1967; Triseliotis 1973; Howe and Feast 2000). Fourth, research reveals that adopted adults who want to make contact, most frequently with their birth mothers, do so largely because information alone cannot satisfy their lingering curiosity. They do not generally report a need to establish lost parental relationships and continue to feel that their adoptive parents fulfil this role. This appears to be the case even where adoptive relationships have proved difficult and unless they have been experienced as extremely traumatic.

To date, Howe and Feast (2000) provide the most recent and complete research data about adopted adults who search for information. They analysed questionnaires completed by 394 adopted adults who had received a relevant service from The Children's Society between 1988 and 1997. Additionally, they were able to identify adopted adults who had never initiated a search. This was achieved through the Society's Intermediary Service, which acted on behalf of birth relatives who were seeking contact with adopted individuals. Information is available for seventy-eight non-searchers who completed a questionnaire. The majority of searchers were placed for adoption in the 1960s and 1970s. We already know something about the characteristics of adopted adults who search for further information and their reasons for doing so. The comparison of searchers and non-searchers provided by Howe and Feast is, however, of particular interest in the context of this discussion. No differences were found between the two groups in relation to perceptions of how openly adoptive parents had discussed adoption, comfort about asking parents for information and how much information was provided. However, significant differences emerged between 60 per cent of non-searchers who thought their adoptive parents had passed on all available information and 50 per cent of searchers who were doubtful about this or thought some information had been withheld. Similarly, only 48 per cent of searchers expressed satisfaction with the information they had been given, compared with 64 per cent of non-searchers. Seventy per cent of searchers compared to only 48 per cent of non-searchers said they wondered why their mothers had placed them for adoption.

Howe and Feast considered whether searchers were distinguishable from non-searchers in relation to feeling different from their adoptive families, feelings of acceptance and belonging and evaluation of their adoptive experience. They found that significantly more non-searchers than searchers expressed no feelings of difference, felt happy about being adopted, felt loved by their adoptive mothers,

expressed feelings of belonging and evaluated their experience of adoption positively. While those describing themselves as black, Asian or of 'mixed heritage'
were significantly more likely to report feeling different from their adoptive
families, they were indistinguishable from other respondents in the extent to which
they felt happy about their adoption and felt loved by their adoptive mothers. There
was a small but non-significant trend for more trans-racially adopted adults
to express feelings that they did not belong to their adoptive families. It should
be noted, however, that 68 per cent of all respondents covering both groups reported
they were happy about being adopted, 78 per cent felt loved by their adopted
mothers and 70 per cent felt they belonged in their adoptive families. Howe and
Feast (2000: 165) conclude:

> It certainly seems to be the case that significantly more searchers than non-
> searchers describe relationships with their adoptive family and their overall
> experience of being adopted with mixed or negative feelings. This finding
> suggests that feeling ambivalent or negative about one's adoption might be
> one factor that motivates some people to search.

Triseliotis (1973) similarly identifies the significance of loving and accepting
adoptive families and a positive adoption experience in differentiating between
adopted adults in his sample who only wanted further information and those
who wanted contact with birth parents. Adopted people who felt they did not belong
and who had experienced adoptive relationships as lacking warmth and closeness
were far more likely to seek contact, most often with their birth mothers. However,
Howe and Feast point out that, expressed as an overall evaluation, 53 per cent of
searchers still felt positively about their adoption experience. Thus, factors
associated with adoptive relationships and family environment play some part
in differentiating between those who choose to search and those who do not, but
cannot provide a complete explanation for variations in searching behaviour. Howe
and Feast (2000: 165) suggest that 'the decision to search is unlikely to be the result
of a single or simple psychological process'. It is more likely to reflect a complex
cluster of motivational factors in individual cases, which are difficult to unravel
into relatively straightforward general causal relationships.

Unfortunately, there is only incomplete information about the number of adopted
adults who want to know more about their background or who plan to contact their
birth families. Such information is collected about adults who were adopted in
England and Wales before 12 November 1975 and who are, therefore, required to
have a counselling interview before being given access to their original birth
records. Numbers of adopted people from this source and those adopted after the
cut-off time who choose to receive counselling from the Family Records Centre
(part of the General Register Office), local authorities or voluntary adoption agencies are recorded by the Office for National Statistics. Its records show that 3,861
adopted adults were counselled in 1990, falling to 2,814 in 1993 and remaining
between 3,644 and 3,224 from 1994 to 2000 (Registrar General 2001: 119). Of
course, many people who are not required to do so under section 26(6) of the 1975

Children Act will not choose to be counselled and any adopted adult who has necessary birth information may apply for a copy of their original birth certificate direct from the Registrar General. The Office for National Statistics will not count these individuals. Triseliotis (2002) suggests that around 37,500 adopted adults, constituting something like half the total number, have sought further background information or contact with their birth families. Howe and Feast (2000: 14) describe the number of adopted people who search as likely to be 'quite high' and refer to the estimate of around 30 to 40 per cent provided by Brodzinsky *et al.* (1992). Ryburn (1992: 82) asserts that in New Zealand, where provision for access to birth records is well advertised, a high proportion of adopted people apply for birth information. He cites Griffith (1991) as estimating that, during five years following implementation of the Adult Adoption Information Act in 1985, around 40 per cent of people adopted by strangers sought access to their birth records.

What are we to glean from all this? Research data about adopted adults seeking further information or birth-family contact relate to those who were adopted at a time when openness remained beyond the vocabulary of placing agencies. They, therefore, had relatively little information about their backgrounds and felt inhibited from raising the topic of adoption within their families. We do know from these studies that adopted people want information about why they were placed for adoption and characteristics that provide a genealogical link with their birth families – shared physical features, common personality traits, and inherited talents and interests. The difficulty is that we do not know how many adopted people live comfortable and well-adjusted lives without this information and have no need or desire to seek it out. Neither do we know how many adopted people, who have not initiated a search, are dissatisfied about their lack of knowledge but feel restrained from searching because of worries about upsetting their adoptive parents, fears about discovering unpalatable information, concerns about unsettling their lives and so on. Howe and Feast (2001: 59) provide some information about their sample of seventy-eight non-searchers. Of interest is the finding that, of this group who had not initiated a search, 42 per cent said they had considered doing so before a birth relative made contact with the Children's Society. Only eight non-searchers refused to have any contact with birth relatives who were trying to get in touch with them. The non-searchers cannot, therefore, be characterised as comprising people who had no interest in their background or birth families. Howe and Feast (2000: 169) respond to these findings by suggesting that 'for the majority of adopted people, questions of identity, genealogical connectedness and the need to have the full story appear to be endemic'. The non-searchers in their sample may have been potential searchers who, for various reasons, remained inactive for the time being. In terms of the relative importance for adopted adults of achieving information and accomplishing contact, it is noteworthy that 85 per cent of the searchers in Howe and Feast's study followed the receipt of information by attempting to effect a reunion with one or more birth relatives. Seventy-five per cent wanted to find their birth mothers.

McWhinnie (1994) thinks advocates for continuing contact, and particularly direct contact, have got it wrong. At the very least, they cannot adequately demonstrate that they have got it right. She argues it is misleading to assert that adopted children need ongoing contact with their birth families on the basis of unrepresentative research samples of adopted adults who choose to search. One of her reasons for caution appears to be that adopted children and adults think of those who brought them up as their 'real' parents. She emphasises the social and emotional construction of identity, arguing that children who grow up in loving and secure adoptive families generally become happy and well-adjusted adults who do not experience any dislocation in their sense of self. This is the picture that tends to emerge from early follow-up studies of adoption when most children grew up without birth-family contact (Witmer *et al.* 1963; Kornitzer 1968; Jaffee and Fanshel 1970; Kadushin 1970; Hoopes *et al.* 1970; Seglow *et al.* 1972). While research indicates that many adopted adults identify closely with their adoptive families, some still search for information about their birth families and go on to locate them. So, it is quite possible for individuals to have close social and emotional ties with their adoptive families but to seek 'genealogical satisfaction' and 'completion' through pursuing contact with their birth families. McWhinnie refers to Craig's (1993) study of young adopted adults, two-fifths of whom indicated they might seek a meeting with birth parents later in order to satisfy their curiosity. Just under a third of the sample expressed no interest in further information or contact and about a fifth appeared to be ambivalent. Using postal questionnaires, Lacey-Smith and Aldgate (1992) followed up twenty-seven adopted adults, aged between 20 and 22, who had been adopted as babies. Of these respondents, 95 per cent said they had not wanted contact with their birth parents while they were growing up and only 15 per cent suggested they would have appreciated *ongoing* information about their birth families. However, around 60 per cent expressed curiosity about their backgrounds and would have liked some material, for example photographs, which would enable them to make links with their genealogy. McWhinnie (1994: 22) cites this study as reporting 'our survey supports the need and wish for background information – it must not be confused with a yearning for contact with the birth family'. Similarly, McWhinnie refers to comments made by adopted people to the Scottish Office consultation on the future of adoption. The consultation paper (Scottish Office 1993: 7.11) remarks: 'The overwhelming majority of adoptees who responded to the Review rejected the concept of continuing contact with their birth parents. They viewed such contact as an unwelcome and unnecessary intrusion into their family life.'

In McWhinnie's (1967) study of fifty-two adopted adults, who were not identified because they were searching for information, only five expressed an interest in tracing their birth mothers. Although many adopted adults in Triseliotis's (1973) sample appear to have been unhappy and confused, he reports that 'the adoptees desired full background information about their origins and genealogy. They maintained that the existence of such material would make it unnecessary for many of them to pursue contact with their natural parents' (p. 149). McWhinnie accepts research findings that indicate the need for adopted children to have full information about their backgrounds and material artefacts to help them fill the 'genealogical gap'. She also accepts that some children, as they grow to adulthood, may want to pursue further information or to arrange meetings with birth-family members. However, McWhinnie most definitely disapproves of general statements, on the basis of limited evidence, to the effect that adopted children should have continuing contact with their birth families because this is the only arrangement that effectively meets their identity needs and thus contributes to their well-being.

Studies of searchers and information about non-searchers, who were adopted twenty to fifty years ago, provide little help in answering two crucial questions. First, would these adopted adults have experienced a need to search if, during child-hood, they had been given full information about their backgrounds in adoptive families where adoption could be easily discussed? Second, under these circum-stances, would information be sufficient to address genealogical issues without a need to contact birth-family members and particularly mothers? In other words, is it necessary to arrange post-adoption contact for children as a response to antic-ipating the information needs expressed by (some) adopted adults? Additionally, most adult research respondents were adopted as babies. Currently, however, contact is likely to be an issue that is considered in relation to looked-after children, most of whom are around 4 or 5 years old when they are placed for adoption. Most of these children will have lived for several years with their birth parents. Many will have experienced abuse and placement change, accompanied by parental opposition to adoption (Ivaldi 1998; Department of Health 2000; Performance and Innovation Unit 2000). While we may draw some general conclusions from the information and contact needs reported by adopted adults, their experiences are notably different from children who are currently being placed for adoption. It is thus difficult to gauge how far these rather different populations will share similar identity issues and to what extent the desire for birth-family contact will be felt by today's adopted children.

Ryburn (1995) throws a little light on information requested by 74 adopted children who had been looked after by local authorities and whose birth parents contested their adoption. The children's mean age at placement was 3½ and, at the time of Ryburn's research, their mean age was 11. Adoptive parents identified children's information needs by completing a postal questionnaire, which asked what kinds of questions children asked about their birth families. Ryburn categorised responses into four groups. First, children asked for factual informa-tion about the material circumstances and relationships in their birth families. Second, questions concerned the health and well-being of birth-family members. Third, children wanted information about themselves and their histories. Fourth, requests for information focused on genealogical issues associated with children's likeness to birth relatives and the clarification of relationships. It was clear from adoptive parents' answers that children emphasised different information needs at various stages of their development and in response to particular circumstances and experiences. Even though these adoptions were completed relatively recently, only thirty-five (47 per cent) of the sixty-seven adopters felt they had sufficient information to answer their children's questions. Ryburn argues that adopted children need continuously updated information about their birth families and that static accomplishments, like photographs and life-story books, cannot meet this requirement. Additionally, adoptive parents still have insufficient information to answer their children's questions. He concludes 'the open exchange of information, which in many instances may most easily be achieved through contact . . . is likely to be a vital factor in adopted children's achievement of a positive sense of identity' (Ryburn 1995: 62). All in all, then, the most effective way to deal with these issues is to arrange continuing post-adoption contact, preferably including direct contact.

There are very little research data about adopted children's perceptions of contact. However, Thomas *et al.* (1999) talked to thirty-eight adopted children, aged between 8 and 15, who had on average lived with their adoptive families for five years, eight months. Of the three children in letter contact and nine children in face-to-face contact with birth parents, six expressed satisfaction with the arrangements. A further five children wanted increased contact with birth mothers and one child was considering a reduction of contact. Twenty-six children had no contact with birth parents and twelve of these wanted to maintain this arrangement. Seven children explicitly rejected the idea of contact but seven children wanted contact to be arranged. Six of seventeen children who were in contact with their siblings wanted more frequent contact. When ten children without sibling contact were asked about this, two expressed a wish to initiate contact. These children's views may change as they grow up. Those without contact may wish to search later on and those with contact may want to extend birth-family relationships through avenues that have been kept open during childhood. However, this study provides equivocal results where many children were apparently satisfied with no contact or explicitly rejected this possibility. Macaskill (2002) discussed their experience of face-to-face contact with thirty-seven children and young people living in permanent family placements, who were aged between 5 and 21 years. They had joined their current families when they were at least 4 years old and had experienced emotional abuse prior to placement. She notes that, although they were all in contact with at least one birth relative, twenty children wanted to establish contact with further family members, most frequently birth mothers. Children generally wanted more contact than had been arranged. The children and young people gave varied reasons for maintaining contact, including feelings of emotional closeness with birth relatives, the need for reassurance about relatives' well-being and access to information about themselves and their histories. However, contact was not always unproblematic or clearly conducive to children's well-being. There were sixty-eight children in Macaskill's study, including thirty-seven whom she interviewed. Of this total she rated only eight children as enjoying unequivocally positive contact. Four children appeared to be indifferent to contact and thirty-nine children reacted ambivalently, expressing anger, sadness and confusion alongside love, relief and pleasure. Macaskill concludes that contact was a negative experience for seventeen children who were rejected, ignored or treated as vehicles for meeting the emotional needs of birth-family members. We cannot tell from Macaskill's discussion whether children's perceptions and experiences of contact were different in relation to placement with long-term foster families or with adoptive families. Fratter's (1996) study of thirteen adopted children and young people with varying types of birth-family contact concluded that children attributed different levels of emotional significance to contact but that they all found it beneficial to some degree.

What we can safely conclude so far is that adopted children generally want to know about the circumstances of their adoption, their birth families and how they connect with their genealogical antecedents. Some adopted people who are unable to access this knowledge or accomplish these connections during childhood seek to do so when they become adults. The quality of relationships and sense of belonging experienced by adopted children as they grow up appears to influence searching behaviour. There also seems to be a relationship between variations in searching, adopted people's satisfaction with information about their background and perceptions about adoptive parents' evasion in withholding information. Research with children who are experiencing contact indicates that some children want and value meetings with their birth families. For some, however, contact can be as painful as it is pleasurable and not all arrangements appear to privilege children's needs over those of adults. Thus far, studies of adopted adults and children do not allow firm conclusions to be drawn about the relative importance of contact versus information for identity development and adjustment, the relative merits of direct (face-to-face) or indirect contact or the conditions under which different kinds of contact might be helpful.

## Further research: the impact of contact on birth and adoptive parents

An alternative way of assessing the benefits of contact is to look for research that studies the impact of contact and its consequences for adoptive parents, children and birth-family members. Much of this work has been carried out in the USA and concentrates on the degree of comfort and satisfaction with contact arrangements expressed by adoptive parents and birth relatives, most frequently parents. In Barth and Berry's (1988) study of 120 adoptive families, 97 per cent of the children had contact with former caregivers or birth relatives, including 42 per cent with foster carers, 27 per cent with birth parents, 32 per cent with birth siblings and 27 per cent with other relatives. Seventeen per cent of adoptive parents found contact to be slightly helpful and 31 per cent said it was very helpful. However, Barth and Berry identified a significant relationship between adopters' perceptions that contact was helpful and their feelings of control over contact arrangements. Nelson's (1985) study of 120 older-child adoptions identified contact with birth relatives in 20 per cent of cases. Fifty per cent of adoptive parents were satisfied with contact arrangements, 37 per cent were ambivalent and only 9 per cent were opposed to contact. Siegal (1993) looked at twenty-one adoptive couples who had experienced 'open' adoption, although the degree of openness varied from an exchange of letters between birth and adoptive parents to ongoing meetings. Much of the direct contact was evidently between birth mothers and adopters and it is unclear how far it included children or how long it continued. None of the adopters regretted agreeing to an open adoption. They all identified advantages associated with their knowledge about birth families' circumstances and characteristics and the provision of detailed and readily accessible information for their children.

In 1993 Berry reported on a questionnaire survey of 1,268 families who had adopted 1,396 children in California. She was interested in identifying adopters' experience of open adoption, which featured a wide variety of arrangements including limited meetings between birth and prospective adoptive parents, post-placement and post-adoption contact of different types between adults, and ongoing direct and indirect contact involving adopted children. The children in Berry's sample were placed for adoption via state agencies, voluntary agencies and independent centres/lawyers, all of which had different practices regarding open adoption. These different arrangements make her analysis rather complicated. In summary, however, Berry found that pre-placement information sharing and post-placement contact were 'fairly common' in her sample and most adoptive parents were 'cautiously comfortable' with post-placement contact. The experience of comfort was significantly related to having an opportunity to plan contact and the implementation of agreed plans. Other factors positively related to adopters' comfort were the absence of child abuse, birth mothers' education, greater 'direct-ness' of contact arrangements, older adoptive mothers and pre-placement meetings between adoptive and birth parents. While trans-racially adopted children enjoyed less contact than others, their adoptive parents were no different from same-race adopters in their degree of comfort and satisfaction with contact. Etter (1993) reports responses from ninety-three adoptive and thirty-six birth parents to questions about their satisfaction and compliance with contact arrangements. The children in this study had been adopted four and a half years before and, in 87 per cent of cases, contact involved direct meetings between adoptive families and birth parents. None of the adoptive parents expressed dissatisfaction with their experience of open adoption and 94 per cent of birth parents said they were satisfied with how open adoption was working. Over 70 per cent of adoptive and birth parents felt satisfied with contact arrangements. Twenty-three of thirty-two adoptive couples interviewed by Gross (1993), where adoptive and birth families had post-placement meetings, were all rated as very satisfied with contact arrangements and their relationships with birth parents. In two cases post-placement meetings had not occurred, but only two adoptive families reported that difficulties with contact had led to their termination. Similarly high levels of satisfaction with contact and comfort with relationships were also identified for the birth-parent sample.

In Britain, Fratter *et al.* (1991) interviewed adoptive parents in twenty-two families experiencing a variety of post-adoption contact arrangements, including face-to-face contact with birth parents. They report that sixteen families felt positively about contact and could identify benefits for themselves and their children. Four years later Fratter (1996) asked these families if she could interview them again. She was able to talk to adoptive parents in eighteen families, and extended the earlier study to include interviews with thirteen children and five birth parents. All the birth parents, and adopters in fifteen families, expressed positive attitudes to contact and said they found it helpful. In New Zealand, Iwanek

(1987) and Dominick (1988) investigated the impact of meetings between adopters and birth mothers. Both studies found that the majority of birth and prospective adoptive parents who met each other experienced the meetings as beneficial. However, these initial meetings characterising open adoption in New Zealand had not necessarily resulted in continued contact for adoptive families. In Dominick's study, only a fifth of adoptive families were still in touch with their children's birth mothers three to four years later and there was very little face-to-face contact.

Studies, particularly from the USA, indicate that various forms of open adoption, including meetings between adoptive families and birth parents, can work positively for all those involved. Not only do most respondents report feeling satisfied and comfortable about contact, but many adoptive parents identify consequential benefits for their children (Siegel 1993; Fratter 1996; Ryburn 1996; Lowe *et al.* 1999). Perceived advantages of contact commonly include maintaining emotionally significant links, access to current information about birth relatives and reassurance about their well-being, retaining a sense of continuity and identity (the importance of 'roots') and avoiding later emotional turmoil through the need to 'search' or to uncover missing information. Some research also suggests contact can have a beneficial effect on the quality of adoptive parenting and adopters' feelings of comfort about contact and birth-family relationships. For example, there is some indication that continuing contact, and particularly face-to-face contact, helps adoptive parents to feel confident about their parenting, more satisfied with contact arrangements and secure in a sense of 'entitlement' to their adopted child (Belbas 1986; Iwanek 1987; Dominick 1988; Berry 1993; Fratter 1996; Sykes 2000). In their study of different openness arrangements, Grotevant and McRoy (1998) found a statistically significant relationship between levels of openness and adoptive parents' anxieties that birth parents might try to reclaim their child. Anxiety was lower and a sense of security higher in 'fully disclosed' adoptions where there was ongoing contact and, in the majority of cases, face-to-face contact between birth mothers and adoptive families. Adopters in relatively closed adoptions based their fear about reclaiming on general impressions and media stories, while those in fully disclosed adoptions were reassured by their personal knowledge of birth parents. Grotevant and McRoy also identified a positive association between fully disclosed adoptions and adopters' feelings of empathy towards their children and birth parents. Adoptive parents in fully disclosed adoptions were also more likely to discuss adoption and birth families with their children during everyday family conversations.

Additionally, research has drawn attention to the negative impact of adoption on the long-term mental health and emotional adjustment of many birth mothers (Winkler and van Keppel 1984; Bouchier *et al.* 1991; Howe *et al.* 1992; Wells 1993; Hughes and Logan 1993). Ongoing information about children's well-being and post-adoption contact of various types can help some birth parents to cope with their sense of loss and to feel positively about their adoption decision (Iwanek 1987; Dominick 1988; Rockel and Ryburn 1988; Howe *et al.* 1992). Research indicates that birth parents do not always want contact and are sensitive to children's needs for stability and security in their adoptive families (Sachdev 1991; Hughes 1995).

## Further research: the impact of contact on children

The way in which different arrangements for openness and post-adoption contact may contribute to children's well-being must be a central issue in decision-making. It is likely that adoptive parents' satisfaction with contact will reflect attitudes to openness, which are helpful to children. However, what we really want to know is how contact impacts on children themselves. We know something, from studies discussed above, about children's desire for contact and their perceptions of its positive and negative consequences. While responsiveness to children's wishes and feelings may contribute to their relative sense of well-being, we cannot assume that contact will necessarily be conducive to healthy development in the longer term. This is why Quinton *et al.* (1997 and 1998) insist that confidence in the benefits of contact is premature. We simply do not know how different forms of contact influence children's intellectual and psychosocial development over time. To proceed with confidence we need the results of longitudinal and comparative studies, which relate measurable aspects of children's development to varying kinds and levels of contact.

Grotevant and McRoy's (1998) research in the USA is the nearest we have to a longitudinal investigation of how different post-adoption openness and contact arrangements affect children's development. They identified 190 adoptive families from thirty-five agencies across the United States. The 171 'target' children who were included in the study had all been adopted before their first birthday and were aged between 4 and 12 years at the first phase of the research. Birth mothers included in the sample numbered 169 and all had voluntarily relinquished their children for adoption. Variables relating to adoptive parents, children and birth mothers were compared in relation to four types of closed/open adoption situations. First, confidential adoptions (sixty-two adoptive families and fifty-two birth mothers) comprised those where no information had been shared between birth and adoptive parents following six months of placement. Second, in time-limited mediated adoptions (seventeen adoptive families and eighteen birth mothers), the agency had passed information between parents but this had stopped before the research. In the third group (fifty-two adoptive families and fifty-eight birth mothers), indirect contact was being maintained via the agency. The fourth group of families (fifty-seven adoptive families and forty-one birth mothers) had 'fully disclosed' adoptions. At the time of the research adoptive parents and birth mothers continued to share information without an intermediary, 'usually' in face-to-face meetings, which were also attended by 86 per cent of the target children. There are, however, possible confounding variables within these groups. For example, almost 50 per cent of children, whose birth and adoptive parents were continuing indirect contact via the agency, were excluded from this information exchange and most of them were not aware of the arrangement. Similarly, the category of 'fully disclosed' adoptions comprised a range of openness forms from occasional letters or telephone calls to several meetings a year.

Research data about the target children are of particular interest in the context of this discussion. Data include children's degree of understanding about adoption, satisfaction with openness, curiosity about birth parents, socio-emotional adjust-ment, self-esteem and sense of identity. Children's satisfaction with the openness of their adoptions did not vary according to openness arrangements, although younger children expressed greater satisfaction. All children across different open-ness groups were curious about their birth parents; their degree of curiosity was unrelated to actual openness or to their perception of openness. The seventy-five children in the sample aged 7½ and over were tested for self-esteem. All showed levels of self-esteem comparable to those of children in the general population and this was not differentially related to families' openness groupings. Grotevant and McRoy (1998: 102) conclude:

> The lack of significant differences for self-esteem, curiosity, satisfaction, and socioemotional adjustment by openness level indicates that the results of this study are not compatible with assertions raised by critics of openness stating that such arrangements will damage children's self esteem and cause con-fusion. *But neither do these findings support the hypothesis that more openness enhances these outcomes.*
>
> (Our emphasis)

At this stage, then, Grotevant and McRoy's study does not indicate that greater openness, including face-to-face contact, contributes to children's well-being or development on a number of dimensions. Their findings may change as they follow these children through adolescence to young adulthood. Given the apparent lack of any significant association between openness levels and children's socio-emotional adjustment, Grotevant and McRoy (Grotevant *et al.* 1999) approached their data from another angle. They undertook a detailed analysis of interview transcripts for twelve sets of adoptive parents and corresponding birth mothers. The adopted children in these families had the highest risk scores for factors thought likely to adversely affect their development. Grotevant *et al.* then rated these 'kin-ship networks' (adoptive parents and birth mothers) according to the nature and quality of their collaboration in respect of contact arrangements and a readiness to respond to children's needs. This sample was very small and demonstrating statistical correlations was thus problematic. However, Grotevant *et al.* did identify a relationship between greater collaboration and better socio-emotional adjustment in the children concerned. It is possible that the attitudes and feelings, which made collaboration difficult for adopters and birth parents, also had a negative impact on children independently of the rating given to the collaborative efforts of their parents. Nevertheless, the research does indicate that adult interactions and rela-tionships bearing on the management of open adoption are likely to affect children's well-being. This suggestion accords with what we know about other family separations where, for example, children's socio-emotional adjustment following divorce tends to be affected more by parental behaviour (levels of collaboration) than it is by the experience of separation *per se* (Schaffer 1990).

So far, Grotevant and McRoy's investigations have identified differences between the attitudes and experiences of adoptive parents and children involved in fully disclosed adoptions compared to ongoing mediated and confidential adoptions. However, to date they have found no differences in children's socio-emotional development in relation to the degree of openness in their adoption. Further clues about the significance of contact for children's well-being might be provided by the relationship, if any, between placement disruption and contact arrangements. Quinton *et al.* (1997 and 1998) reviewed the evidence on this front, concentrating on contact with birth parents. Research by Borland *et al.* (1991) and Barth and Berry (1988) failed to identify a significant relationship between ongoing contact and placement stability. Holding constant other variables associated with placement disruption, such as age at placement, Fratter *et al.* (1991) did demonstrate a statistically significant association between increased placement stability and ongoing contact with birth parents. However, at the point of data analysis the sample children had been in placement for between eighteen months and six and a half years, thus representing different time periods over which disruptions could occur and during which parental contact was maintained. Quinton *et al.* (1997) suggest we need a more detailed account of the statistical analyses employed by Fratter and her colleagues before reaching any conclusions about the protective role played by parental contact. We would add that, while statistically significant correlations are important in directing attention to relationships between variables, they have relatively little explanatory power. In this sense, a statistical association between contact and placement stability requires supplementing with data about the frequency and reliability of contact, how it is managed and arranged, parental attitudes to children's placements and the relationship between parents, children and permanent carers. Making contact arrangements is problematic in *individual cases* if we do not understand how and why contact may contribute to placement stability.

## Conclusion: how much do we know about the benefits of continuing contact?

Studies of adopted adults who search for information or who seek contact with their birth relatives tell us something about the significance of genealogical information, the need to complete a sense of self and the importance of developing a narrative that locates identity in a genetic and social context. Evidential guidance about current practice and contact arrangements is largely provided by an assortment of small-scale studies that employ different methodological approaches. The studies ask different questions of different respondents, include a variety of often unspecified contact arrangements, involve a range of birth relatives, refer to children of widely varying ages and backgrounds and often fail to differentiate between birth parents' agreement with or opposition to adoption. Additionally, many studies from the USA and New Zealand rely on samples of birth parents and adopters involved in the adoption of children who were voluntarily relinquished as infants. It is arguable that attitudes to contact and the way children experience contact arrangements may differ between situations where children are voluntarily relinquished as infants and where they are placed for adoption when older because of abusive or inadequate parenting and in the face of parental opposition. Furthermore, some benefits attributed to openness and contact such as adoptive parents' empathic attitudes, acknowledgement of 'difference' and a sense of security in the parenting role may not develop as a consequence of contact. It may be that people with these characteristics are more willing to co-operate with contact arrangements in the first instance. Bearing these difficulties in mind, we think it is still legitimate to draw some very tentative conclusions from available research. First, there appears to be increasing professional support for post-adoption contact and many adoptive parents are willing to facilitate this. Second, it is possible to maintain helpful contact with birth parents notwithstanding their opposition to adoption. Third, many adopters experience contact as beneficial for their children and for themselves and express satisfaction with contact arrangements. Fourth, some adopted children may value contact and want it to continue. Fifth, ongoing contact does not seem to interfere with adoptive parents' sense of security or their perceived status as parents and it may actually enhance these feelings.

Quinton *et al.* (1997) must be correct in their argument that we do not yet have sufficient information about the long-term consequences of different types of contact arrangements, or of no contact, for children's development. However, they are willing to concede that post-adoption contact 'can work amicably' and that, all other things being equal, contact between children and emotionally important adults is of some significance for children's well-being. Their purpose in disputing professed certainty about the benefits of contact is to clarify the evidential basis which informs this position 'in circumstances where stable, nurturing relationships with birth parents have usually not been part of the child's experience' (Quinton *et al.* 1997: 394). We have noted the problems associated with reaching firm and unequivocal conclusions on the basis of available research. For adults and children who want contact and identify it as beneficial in various ways, there are others with different stories to tell. The outstanding problem is that we remain relatively unclear about the *conditions* under which contact is experienced as beneficial by those involved and which are likely to differentially influence long-term outcomes for children.

Quinton *et al.* (1997) do not underestimate the methodological difficulties associated with the kind of longitudinal studies they recommend. There are, indeed, enormous problems in trying to identify significant causal relationships between contact arrangements and outcomes. The impact of contact cannot be evaluated simply by categorising arrangements for some or no contact and relating these categories to measures of children's socio-emotional development and birth and adoptive parents' attitudes. When Grotevant, McRoy and their associates began working with their sample, which we have discussed above, they started with three categories of contact. However, they found that these were inadequate to convey respondents' experience of contact and enhanced their categorisation to include five groups. Further analysis revealed additional differences between contact arrangements and thirty-three sub-categories were therefore introduced to reflect these distinctions (McRoy 1991: 103). The final categorisation distinguishes between the amount and nature of communication between birth and adoptive parents, the period over which information sharing extends, the direction in which information is conveyed, the inclusion of photographs and telephone calls, and provision of identifying and non-identifying information. Distinctions are also made between the type and frequency of face-to-face meetings. Thus, any study that purports to relate contact to outcomes must control for a wide variety of arrangements that may differentially impact on birth relatives, adoptive parents and children. Other significant factors, which may influence outcome include the quality of adoptive family relationships, the child's pre-placement experience and socio-emotional functioning, birth and adoptive parents' attitudes to contact, the quality and reliability of contact and birth parents' reactions to adoption. Additionally, the nature and frequency of contact and participants' experience may change over time. Children's development and adults' attitudes therefore require measurement at intervals until children reach adulthood.

It appears that practitioners are continuing to make arrangements for post-adoption contact in advance of the kind of research that might effectively inform their decisions. They are, furthermore, supported by a vociferous band of advocates who think that ongoing contact is in children's long-term best interests. Under these conditions, exploratory studies such as our own may help to focus attention on factors that influence how adoptive parents, children and birth relatives experience contact arrangements, particularly where children are not voluntarily relinquished as infants. Qualitative data can help us understand the processes and interactions that contribute to the impact of contact and the way it is perceived by those involved.

## Summary

- Adoption is now increasingly characterised by arrangements for some form of post-adoption contact. However, while some researchers and practitioners are convinced that contact (and preferably face-to-face contact) contributes to children's well-being, others argue that there is insufficient evidence about its long-term effects on children's development to support such confidence.
- Research indicates that adopted children generally want to know about the circumstances of their adoption, their birth families and how they connect with their genealogical antecedents. Some adopted people who are unable to access this knowledge or accomplish these connections during childhood seek to do so when they become adults. There appears to be some relationship between searching for birth relatives, usually birth mothers, unhappy experiences of adoption and a belief that adoptive parents have withheld information.
- Although there is relatively little research on adopted children's perceptions, it is evident that many children want and value contact. However, studies indicate that contact is not always unproblematic and may involve painful feelings and memories for children who, nonetheless, want its continuation.
- Many adopters experience contact as beneficial for themselves and their children and express satisfaction with contact arrangements. It is possible to establish helpful contact with birth parents notwithstanding contested adoption

proceedings. Post-adoption contact does not seem to interfere with adoptive parents' sense of security or their sense of 'entitlement' to their children and may actually enhance these feelings.

- Thus far, research has not provided unequivocal evidence about the conditions under which particular forms of post-adoption contact are likely to be experienced as beneficial by adopters, children and birth relatives. In any event qualitative features of interaction, communication, relationships, attitudes and so on will influence individuals' experience of contact. Decisions about contact must therefore be made in relation to the needs, characteristics and circumstances of particular children and their families rather than in response to general evidential rules or ideological commitment.

# 3   Policy, law and openness in adoption

## Policy issues: openness and access to information

As we have noted, legislation in 1926 for England and Wales and 1930 for Scotland was designed to provide legal recognition of adoption and to clarify the respective rights and legal status of children, birth parents and adopters following an adoption order. Law's initial intervention was thus concerned with identifying the conditions under which an adoption order could be made, the necessity for parental consent and grounds for dispensing with consent and the legal consequences of adoption. Policy-makers had little inclination to interfere with arrangements between those most centrally involved in making adoption arrangements. The Tomlin Committee, which submitted three reports (Tomlin 1925, 1926a and 1926b) recommending a legal framework for adoption, warned against practice that sought to introduce secrecy into adoptive relationships. The Committee commented that complete secrecy was 'unnecessary' and 'objectionable' and that adoption societies should not 'deliberately seek to fix a gulf between the child's past and future' (Tomlin 1925: 8). Concern about unregulated practice by adoption societies prompted the government to establish the Horsburgh Committee in 1936 (Horsburgh Committee 1937). This committee disapproved of practice which attempted to conceal the identity of prospective adopters from birth parents. It investigated allegations that secrecy was necessary to stop birth parents interfering in the lives of adoptive families but was satisfied that such concerns were unfounded. The Committee saw no reason to withdraw birth parents' rights to have 'an opportunity to satisfy themselves personally as to the suitability of the prospective adopters and as to all other matters with which the court is concerned' (Horsburgh Committee 1937: 22). At this time, however, policy considerations focused on the residual rights of birth parents and not on the needs or rights of adopted people for access to information about their birth families. The Adoption Act of 1950 consolidated legislative change and established the principle that secrecy and anonymity should characterise relationships between the parties to adoption.

In 1953 the Hurst Committee (Hurst Committee 1954) was appointed to review the appropriateness of adoption policy and existing law. The Committee accepted evidence arguing that, as in Scotland, adopted people in England and Wales should be able to access information about their birth parentage. It said:

A number of witnesses in England thought that the adopted person has a right to this information and expressed the view that it is not in the interests of adopted people to be permanently precluded from satisfying their natural curiosity.

(p. 53)

However, due to 'practical difficulties' the Hurst Committee did not recommend making the law in England and Wales consistent with provisions, allowing access to birth records, in the Adoption of Children (Scotland) Act 1930. Instead, it suggested that on reaching the age of twenty-one, adopted adults should have the right to obtain a full copy of their adoption order from the court. This document would include their original names and identify their birth parent(s), thus providing necessary information for obtaining a copy of their birth certificate. The Committee recommended that existing arrangements in Scotland for access to birth information should remain unchanged, except for raising the age allowing access from seventeen to twenty-one. None of the Committee's suggestions in this regard were implemented in the subsequent Adoption Act of 1958.

It took over ten years before policy attention was again directed at the issue of access to information, when the Houghton Committee was set up in 1969 (Houghton Committee 1972) to consider whether any changes were required in adoption legislation. Although from the Houghton Committee's perspective access to birth records was 'not a major issue', the Committee recognised its significance in terms of changing adoption practice and the relative rights of birth parents and adopted adults. Its first report (Houghton Committee 1970) was equivocal about legislating for a right of access to birth records, acknowledging the need for greater openness in adoption while being cautious about the potential consequences of providing *identifying* information about birth parents. However, having heard further representations and evidence from Triseliotis's research on the Scottish system (Triseliotis 1973), the Houghton Committee was eventually persuaded to recommend a change in the law:

> The weight of evidence as a whole was in favour of freer access to background information, and this accords with our wish to encourage greater openness about adoption. We take the view that on reaching the age of majority an adopted person should not be denied access to his original birth records. We therefore recommend that all adopted adults in England and Wales, whenever adopted, should in the future be permitted to obtain a copy of their original birth entry, and that in Scotland the age at which access to original birth records is permitted should similarly be 18, instead of 17 as at present.
>
> (Houghton Committee 1972: 85)

Parliamentary debate on the Houghton Committee's recommendations, which finally informed section 26 in the 1975 Children Act and section 51 in the 1976 Adoption Act, was still much concerned about birth parents' rights. Prior to new legislation, birth parents made their decisions about adoption on the understanding that their anonymity would be preserved. As is now well known, the Children Act 1975 accommodated this problem by incorporating in section 26(6) the requirement for compulsory counselling when anyone adopted before the implementation of section 26, in November 1976, applied to the Registrar General for access to their birth records. Anyone adopted after 26 November 1976 could exercise a choice about whether to use the counselling service. Thus far, the right of access to information was one way and was accorded only to adopted adults.

Schedule 10, paragraph 21 of the Children Act 1989 inserted section 51A into the 1976 Adoption Act requiring the Registrar General to set up and keep a register to be known as the Adoption Contact Register. As long as they met certain conditions, adopted adults could have their name and address recorded under Part 1 of the register and birth relatives wishing to make contact could have the same details recorded under Part 2. Relatives were defined as 'any person (other than an adoptive relative) who is related to the adopted person by blood (including half blood) or marriage'. Where the Registrar General identified a match between entries in Parts 1 and 2 of the register, access to information was again one way – details of a relative's entry were sent to the adopted person. Section 80 of the Adoption and Children Act 2002 confirms earlier arrangements in respect of the Adoption Contact Register but section 80(6) states that decisions about the disclosure of information to people entered in Parts 1 and 2 of the register will be governed by Regulations. Explanatory notes to the 2002 Act suggest that Regulations may provide only for passing birth relatives' details to adopted adults and not vice versa. The National Organisation for the Counselling of Adoptees and Parents (NORCAP), established in 1982, has campaigned tirelessly for a more active intermediary service for adopted adults and birth relatives who indicate a wish to obtain information about each other or to initiate contact. During the Adoption and Children Bill's passage through Parliament, NORCAP argued that the Adoption Contact Register represents only a passive acknowledgement of birth family links broken through adoption. NORCAP supported placing intermediary services on a statutory footing to facilitate safe and mutually acceptable arrangements for the disclosure of information between birth relatives and adopted adults.

Issues about the relative rights of adopted people and birth relatives to obtain information, and particularly identifying information, about each other have concerned policy-makers since 1954 when the Hurst Committee first challenged the aura of secrecy that had come to characterise adoption. The Adoption and Children Act 2002 sets out to resolve these issues. However, the Act's attempt to identify and protect different individuals' rights has resulted in rather complicated proposals governing access to information. Section 56 of the Adoption and Children Act indicates that Regulations will prescribe the information adoption agencies must keep about a person's adoption. This information will be known as 'section 56 information'. The definition of 'protected information' under section 57(3) of the Act includes three types of information. These are, first, 'section 56 information', which identifies or enables the identification of an adopted or other person; second, information obtained by the agency from the Registrar General, which would enable an adopted person to obtain a certified copy of his or her birth record; and third, information about an entry in the Adoption Contact Register relating to an adopted person. Sections 57 to 62 of the Adoption and Children Act detail the conditions under which 'protected' and other information held by adoption agencies may be disclosed to various people. However, section 57(5) states that where there is a prescribed agreement to which the adoption agency is a party, the restrictions on disclosure of 'protected information' do not apply. The Explanatory Notes to the Act clarify that this section 'is intended to allow agreement between the adoption agency, the adoptive parents and the birth parents for the sharing of protected information' (paragraph 167) so that post-adoption contact and other ways of achieving openness can be arranged. An adoption agency may disclose section 56 information, other than 'protected information', to any person 'in accordance with prescribed arrangements' under section 58(2).

Under section 60(2)(a) of the Act, adopted adults have a right to receive information from an agency that would enable them to obtain a copy of their birth record unless the agency obtains an order from the High Court allowing it to refuse this request. Section 51 of the Adoption Act 1976 previously gave adults, who were adopted after 26 November 1976, the right to obtain this information direct from the Registrar General without the intervention of an adoption agency. Section 60(4) also gives adopted adults the right to receive from the court, which made the adoption order, a copy of prescribed documents providing they do not contain 'protected information'. Under section 60(2)(b), an adoption agency must, if requested to do so, provide an adopted adult with any prescribed information that it has given to the adoptive parent(s). Sections 61 and 62 cover the powers and duties of adoption agencies when any person applies to them for 'protected information' about an adult or child. An adoption agency may use its discretion to decide whether to proceed with such an application. If it does proceed, it must take all reasonable steps to obtain the views of the person (and any parent or guardian of a child) about whom 'protected information' has been requested concerning the disclosure of that information to the applicant. When deciding whether to disclose the information that is sought, the agency must consider the subject's views as above and the welfare of any adopted person who is involved. If information is requested about an adopted child, the child's welfare must be the agency's paramount consideration. These arrangements provide a statutory intermediary service between those seeking 'protected information' and those about whom information is sought and they are responsive to criticism of the previous legal framework mounted by organisations like NORCAP. Birth relatives will be able to proactively request 'protected information' about adopted children or adults instead of being powerless to act. Similarly, adopted adults will be able to make enquiries about 'protected information' not covered by their right to information under section 60(2) of the Adoption and Children Act and adoptive parents may apply for information on their own behalf or for their adopted child. These sections of the Adoption and Children Act will apply only to adoptions finalised after implementation of the Act. Arrangements for access to information for people adopted before implementation of sections 56 to 65 are covered by section 98 of the Adoption and Children Act. Section 98 refers to Regulations that will make provision for helping adopted adults to obtain information about their adoption and facilitating contact between adopted persons and their relatives.

Sections in the Adoption and Children Act governing the disclosure of 'protected information' tread a fine line between rights to information and rights to privacy and anonymity for both adopted people and their birth families. The provisions have attracted critical comment on the grounds that they discriminate against adopted children and vest considerable discretion in adoption agencies. Although section 58(2) of the Act allows an adoption agency to provide 'section 56 information' (other than 'protected information') to any person, presumably including children, this is at the agency's discretion. Any application for 'protected information' would be governed by the adoption agency's discretion under sections 61 and 62 of the Act. Children do not then have any *rights* to information about their adoption, history or birth family. Van Bueren (1995) argues that adopted children have suffered a 'history of discrimination' because of their lack of entitlement to information about their backgrounds. She suggests that policy-makers should re-think the balance between birth parents' rights to privacy and anonymity and adopted children's and adults' rights to identifying information. Rights, however, are defined and enforced within a social-policy context and occasionally even apparently absolute rights may legitimately be violated because of wider policy issues. For example, the rights of adopted adults to obtain information from their original birth records under section 26 of the 1975 Children Act and section 51 of the 1976 Adoption Act have been curtailed in individual cases. In *R v Registrar General ex parte Smith* [1991] 2 QB 393, the Court of Appeal upheld the Registrar General's refusal to divulge birth-record information to an adopted adult because of a demonstrable danger that the birth mother might be physically harmed if she was traced. The Gaskin case (*Gaskin v UK (Access to Personal Files)* (1990) 12 EHRR 36), decided by the European Court of Human Rights, has also attracted attention with reference to conditions that should govern access to information. Mr Gaskin had spent most of his life in local-authority care and wanted access to the authority's records about his background. His request was refused and this decision was upheld in the domestic courts. The European Court found that Article 8(1) of the European Convention on Human Rights (respect for privacy and family life) protected Mr Gaskin's right to be given the information he required. It commented that applicants in Mr Gaskin's situation 'have a vital interest, protected by the Convention, in receiving the information necessary to know and to understand their childhood and early development' (paragraph 49). However, as in other circumstances where Article 8(1) is relevant, a breach of the right may be justified under conditions set out in Article 8(2). The European Court of Human Rights did not attribute absolute rights to individuals like Mr Gaskin. Judicial decisions about whether to protect or breach the right of access to information should be informed by any public interest considerations that argue against disclosure and the likely effects of disclosure on third parties and applicants (Swindells *et al.* 1999: 201). Additionally, the Court made it clear it would have considered things differently if Mr Gaskin had been a minor when he was seeking access to information held by the local authority. Issues concerning protection and welfare must inform judicial decisions in the context of children's rights. Advocates for post-adoption contact might argue that ongoing contact between adopted children and their birth families could effectively render this moral and legal debate, and its associated emotional costs, redundant for future generations.

## Policy issues: post-adoption contact

Since the Hurst Committee in 1954 first identified adopted persons' access to information as a policy issue, this aspect of 'openness' has continued to exercise the minds of policy-makers and legislators. However, since the early 1990s post-adoption contact has emerged as a further bone of contention. Advocates for post-adoption contact want to see the development of a policy and legislative framework that supports and enforces continuing contact when this is considered to be in a child's best interests. They consider it unsatisfactory to rely on social-work practice to promote contact and adopters' willingness to maintain it. The Interdepartmental Working Group (1992), which conducted the Review of Adoption Law, appears to be the first policy review body to have formally considered the issue of contact and adoption. It was furnished with background papers on research (Thoburn 1990) and on international perspectives (France 1990) which referred to the significance of contact for children and the common practice of open adoption, particularly in New Zealand and the USA. The Working Group wanted to introduce a firm policy position to ensure that a child's need for ongoing contact was considered at an appropriate time and arrangements for contact were protected if this was deemed to be necessary for a child's well-being. It noted the importance of considering existing and future contact arrangements at the time of an adoption hearing. The Working Group suggested a contact order might be helpful in lending weight to already agreed post-adoption contact and, in exceptional circumstances, might have a place in enforcing contact where agreement could not be reached. Reference to a contact order here means an order made by the court under section 8 of the Children Act 1989. While it has been possible for courts to enforce contact by attaching a condition to an adoption order under section 12(6) of the 1976 Adoption Act, the Interdepartmental Working Group considered that the use of this section was inappropriate. In any event, when implemented, the Adoption and Children Act 2002 will supersede the 1976 Act.

Grasping the nettle, the Working Group made the following recommendations about contact. First, agencies should have a duty, when considering adoption, to consult all relevant individuals (including the child) and to take their views and wishes into account. This would include their views and wishes about continuing contact. Second, any adoption legislation should re-affirm the court's power to make an order for contact under section 8 of the 1989 Children Act alongside an adoption order. Third, the court should have a specific duty to consider making a contact order when hearing an application for adoption. Under these conditions the issue of contact would have to be explicitly addressed by the agency and by any court dealing with an adoption application. The following White Paper (Secretary of State for Health 1993) acknowledged that making arrangements for post-adoption contact was becoming more common and linked this practice to the older age at which children were placed for adoption. While recognising that continuing direct contact might be important for children and birth parents, the White Paper was clear that adoptive parents' views should carry greater weight in any decision about contact. However, the White Paper appeared to respond to the Interdepartmental Working Group's recommendations when it stated 'by regulation, the Government intends to ensure that the courts and adoption agencies will assess the most suitable arrangements for contact between the birth family and the child after his adoption' (paragraph 4.17). The White Paper, and the subsequent Adoption Bill of March 1996, became redundant when the Conservatives lost the general election and the process of adoption law reform had to begin all over again.

Meanwhile the Adoption Law Reform Group, comprising several organisations which were collectively promoting new adoption legislation, kept up the pressure for developing policy on post-adoption contact. The Group pointed out that 'existing law nowhere explicitly acknowledges the changes in practice that have taken place in recent years' (Adoption Law Reform Group 2000: 5) to the extent that some form of post-adoption contact is now commonly arranged. Reflecting the 1992 Interdepartmental Working Group's recommendations, the Adoption Law Reform Group suggested:

> Courts and agencies should be required, when arranging an adoption or considering an application for an adoption order, to consider the significance for the child of his or her existing relationships, and whether and to what extent these can or should be affirmed by an agreement held on the court record, or, if absolutely necessary, by an order for continuing contact. Agencies should be required to facilitate or provide mediation services to assist with contact.

The Prime Minister's Review of Adoption (Performance and Innovation Unit 2000) and the following White Paper (Secretary of State for Health 2000) paid relatively little attention to post-adoption contact. Practice issues largely attracted the Performance and Innovation Unit's attention. It recommended the provision of guidance possibly as part of National Standards, the inclusion of contact in a local authority's duty to provide post-adoption support, joint training for social workers and guardians *ad litem* (now children's guardians), and judicial training about contact. In the White Paper contact issues were consigned to two paragraphs (6.42 and 6.43) where the government acknowledged that birth-family links may be important to children and that this area of practice should be covered by National Adoption Standards.

The Adoption and Children Act 2002 provides an indication of government's response to the considerable pressure for policy and legislative recognition of post-adoption contact. It reflects a substantial development of policy thinking from that expressed in the Prime Minister's Review of Adoption, the White Paper and the October 2001 Adoption and Children Bill. The Act sets out conditions under which an agency is authorised to place a child for adoption. These conditions are that either each parent or guardian has given their consent to placement or a court has made a placement order. Placement orders may only be made in respect of children who are already subject to care orders or where the grounds for a care order under section 31(2) of the Children Act 1989 are met. Additionally, placement orders may be made where a child has no parent or guardian. The necessary consent must be forthcoming or must be dispensed with by the court. When an agency is authorised to place a child for adoption any provisions for contact under the Children Act 1989 cease to apply, but an application for contact may be made under section 26 of the Adoption and Children Act. Additionally, when making a placement order, a court may make any provision for contact without having an application before it. However, section 26(5) makes it clear that an application for a contact order under section 8 of the Children Act may still be made when it is heard together with an adoption application. It is important to note that section 27(4) of the Adoption and Children Act lays an express duty on courts to consider arrangements, which the agency has made or proposes to make for contact between the child and 'any person', before making a placement order. The court hearing an application for a placement order must also invite parties to the proceedings to comment on any contact arrangements.

At the stage of considering a placement order, the Adoption and Children Act thus lays considerable emphasis on directing judicial attention to arrangements for contact. However, contact arrangements will not routinely attract judicial scrutiny at this stage where parents have agreed to placement for adoption and the grounds for a placement order do not apply. Crucially, the Act is responsive to calls for contact arrangements to be explicitly considered when an adoption order is made. Section 46(6) states:

> Before making an adoption order, the court must consider whether there should be arrangements for allowing any person contact with the child; and for that purpose the court must consider any existing or proposed arrangements and obtain any views of the parties to the proceedings.

Courts may also be encouraged to consider the importance of continuing contact by reference to a modified 'welfare checklist' similar to that found in section 1(3) of the 1989 Children Act. Here, whenever a court or adoption agency is 'coming to a decision relating to the adoption of a child' it must have regard, among other matters, to the child's ascertainable wishes and feelings considered in the light of his or her age and understanding. It must also consider the child's relationship with relatives or other significant people, 'the likelihood of any such relationship continuing and the value to the child of its doing so' and the wishes and feelings of relatives and others regarding the child. The court must always consider the range of powers available to it under the newly implemented Act and under the Children Act 1989 – including, of course, its ability to make a contact order under section 8 of the Children Act. The Adoption and Children Act should please advocates of post-adoption contact who want to see a stronger legislative lead on judicial consideration of contact arrangements at the time an adoption order is made. However, the introduction of sections regarding contact into adoption legislation may not result in more extensive legal protection of post-adoption contact arrangements. As Harris-Short (2001: 417) remarks, courts are already able to make a contact order alongside an adoption order:

> The problem does not lie with the court's ability to make the appropriate orders, but with its firmly entrenched resistance to doing so. Without much stronger guidance from the legislature as to the desirability of post-adoption contact it is highly unlikely that this resistance will be broken down, particularly if the adoptive parents are opposed.

Policy emphasises practice discretion concerning contact arrangements, although this will now be subject to judicial consideration when courts hear applications for placement or adoption orders. The National Adoption Standards for England (Department of Health 2001b) provide instructions about how agencies are to exercise their discretion. Adoption plans 'will include details of the arrangements for maintaining links (including contact) with birth parents, wider birth family members and other people who are significant' to children (paragraph A:11). Adoptive parents will be involved in discussions about how they can best maintain any links, including contact. Where the maintenance of ongoing links is considered to be in a child's best interests, birth-family members will be engaged in discussions about how best to achieve this and may be given practical or financial support to help them work to agreed plans. It should be noted here that the Department of Health's reference to 'adoptive parents' appears to include people who have been approved by an agency rather than those who have been granted an adoption order. However, the implication in the National Adoption Standards is that, through discussion with adoptive parents and birth-family members, a constructive agreement will emerge and contact arrangements will be maintained. This approach fails to consider possible responses where adopters are opposed to links or contact or where they withdraw their co-operation after an adoption order is made. Those who advocate greater judicial involvement in contact decisions argue that courts should be more willing to make contact orders at the point of adoption, to enforce or protect contact arrangements against future uncertainty. They also point out that, without an order, birth-family members are relatively powerless to insist on contact if adopters employ their status as the child's legal parents to stop or reduce agreed arrangements.

## Judicial intervention in contact arrangements

Courts can make a contact order under section 8 of the Children Act 1989. A contact order is defined as 'an order requiring the person with whom a child lives, or is to live, to allow the child to visit or stay with the person named in the order, or for that person and the child otherwise to have contact with each other'. Section 11(7) of the Children Act gives the court wide powers to add conditions to a contact order or to specify detailed arrangements for its implementation. Section 10 of the

Act identifies those categories of people who have a right to apply for a contact order, including a child's parents or guardians. Those who do not have a right to apply must, in the first instance, seek the court's leave to make an application. Additionally, in any family proceedings, which includes adoption proceedings, the court may make a contact order on its own initiative if it thinks it is in the child's best interests to do so. Courts have the power to enforce contact orders through fining or imprisoning a person who breaches an order.

Ryburn (1997a and 1997b) argues that judicial attitudes to contact issues following divorce and separation reflect five working principles that are equally relevant in cases of post-adoption contact. These concern the child's right to contact, the benefits of contact for children's well-being, the necessity of enforcing contact, the recognition that long-term benefits will accrue over short-term distress and the importance of establishing contact with a non-custodial parent without delay. In his view, therefore, post-adoption contact should attract a judicial approach that is consistent with the imposition and enforcement of contact arrangements following divorce. However, it should be noted that the Advisory Board on Family Law (2002), reporting to the Lord Chancellor, suggests that courts should play a more limited role in resolving contact disputes between separating and divorcing parents. The Board (2002: 116) recommends:

> The Lord Chancellor's Department should fund additional facilities for resolving contact disputes by negotiation, conciliation and mediation. Whilst there is plainly a role for the court in resolving contact issues, there is a widespread perception that such disputes are better addressed outside the court system. There is a widespread feeling that an application to the court should be the last resort.

There are, however, distinct differences between judicial attitudes towards contact in divorce and adoption proceedings, despite the fact that both situations involve the child's separation from a parent or other family members who may be emotionally important to them. It is necessary to grasp the particular character of adoption to understand why this is the case. Contact issues in divorce involve disputed arrangements for children to maintain contact with a non-resident parent where both parents retain parental responsibility. On adoption, birth parents cease to have parental responsibility and have no legal status in relation to their child. Adoption creates new parents. It acts to transfer legal, social and emotional responsibility for children from birth to adoptive parents. In its review of adoption law, the Interdepartmental Working Group (1992: 3.6) emphasised the significance of adoption:

> Adoption in its present form is an extremely important step in a child's life, which determines his or her identity and family relationships throughout life. It is essential that adoption is regarded not as a means of determining with whom a child is to live, but as a way of making a child legally part of a new family and severing any legal relationships with the birth family. It should

stand apart from other orders, not in such a way that it is thought of as a superior option but so there are no doubts as to its special features.

This understanding of adoption has two important consequences for judicial thinking about contact. First, if post-adoption contact is not agreed prior to adoption or agreements are subsequently broken, birth parents do not have a right to apply for the initiation or variation of contact under section 10 of the Children Act 1989. This is because they are classed as 'former parents' once an adoption order is made. A parent or other birth relative will therefore have to overcome a prior obstacle in the form of an application for leave (the court's permission) to make a contact application. Second, courts have been unwilling to interfere with adoptive parents' exercise of their parental responsibility or to attach conditions to an adoption order. In *Re V (A Minor) (Adoption: Dispensing with Agreement)* [1987] 2 FLR 89, Oliver LJ commented:

> The whole purpose of an adoption order is to transfer to the adopters the control over the upbringing of the adopted child and the power of making all decisions as to his future, and to impose on that some limitation on the way in which the adopters' rights are to be exercised is, in effect a contradiction of the terms of s. 8(1) of the Children Act 1975, which provides that, 'An adoption order is an order vesting the parental rights and duties relating to the child in the adopters . . .'
>
> (p. 104)

Oliver LJ accepted, however, that there might be occasions when a child's welfare required post-adoption contact with a birth parent. He made it clear in this context that any question of contact must recognise the adopters' right to exercise their discretion as the child's legal parents. Otherwise the imposition of conditions on an adoption order would be 'repugnant to the notion of adoption'. *Re C (A Minor) (Adoption Order: Conditions)* [1988] 2 FLR 159 was a case involving post-adoption contact between siblings, which was appealed to the House of Lords. In reviewing established case law on adoption and access, Lord Ackner confirmed that the court had power to make an adoption order with conditions. He was also clear that:

> These cases rightly stress that in normal circumstances it is desirable that there should be a complete break, but that each case has to be considered on its own particular facts. No doubt the court will not, except in the most exceptional case, impose terms or conditions as to access to members of the child's natural family to which the adopting parents do not agree. To do so would be likely to create a potentially frictional situation which would be hardly likely to safeguard or promote the welfare of the child.

Later cases confirmed this approach to adoption. For example, in *Re S (A Minor) (Blood Transfusion: Adoption Order Conditions)* [1994] 2 FLR 416, Staughton LJ commented that the imposition of conditions on adoptive parents should not become common practice. He said 'the best thing for the child in the ordinary way is that he or she should become as near as possible the lawful child of the adopting parents'. *Re T (Adoption: Contact)* [1995] 2 FLR 251 concerned an appeal by adoptive parents against a contact order under section 8 of the Children Act 1989, which was made alongside the adoption order. The child in question had ongoing contact with her older sister and it was agreed that this should continue after adoption. At least annual meetings between the child and her birth mother were also agreed, although the mother indicated that she would like more frequent contact. The adopters argued that a contact order was unnecessary and that they should retain control over contact arrangements. In this case the Court of Appeal agreed and set aside the order for contact. Two main strands of reasoning informed the court's judgment. Section 1(5) of the Children Act 1989 states that where the court is considering making an order under the Act, it should not make an order 'unless it considers that doing so would be better for the child than making no order at all'. In the Court of Appeal's view, the adoptive parents had already undertaken to allow post-adoption contact. An order was unnecessary in this situation where the parties could effectively maintain contact arrangements through mutual trust. The second theme in the court's thinking relates to the nature of adoption and the preferred autonomy of adoptive families. Butler-Sloss LJ said 'in my judgment the prevalence and finality of adoption and the importance of letting the new family find its own feet ought not to be threatened in any way by an order in this case' (p. 544). So, unless there are clearly exceptional circumstances, courts will not make a contact order in opposition to adopters' wishes. Equally, however, courts are unlikely to make an order where adopters agree to contact. Judicial reasoning also doubts that adoption is appropriate where frequent post-adoption contact is envisaged. Oliver LJ expressed his unease in *Re V*, above, that frequent contact was not designed only to keep the birth mother's memory alive and to help the child develop an adequate sense of identity but would also strengthen and develop an existing relationship. He also questioned whether the mother would be able to conceal from the child her wish to have him home. Oliver LJ said:

> Once it is found, however, that regular and frequent access, inevitably maintaining and strengthening the family ties between the child and his mother and her other children, is so conducive to the welfare of the child that provision has to be made for it in the adoption order as the underlying basis on which the order is made at all, I find it difficult to reconcile that with the avowed purpose of the adoption of extinguishing any parental rights or duties in the natural parent.
>
> (p. 98)

More recently, *Re B (Adoption Order)* [2001] 2 FLR 26 concerned a child, who was subject to a care order, and who had enjoyed frequent contact with his father and paternal relatives while placed with his foster mother. The child's father applied for a residence order, but later agreed that a residence order should be made in favour of the foster mother. However, the local authority considered adoption to be in the child's best interests and encouraged the foster mother to apply for an adoption order. It was agreed that post-adoption contact would comprise at least monthly meetings between the child and his father. The birth mother agreed to adoption and the court dispensed with the father's consent and made an adoption order. The father appealed and the Court of Appeal found that the frequency and extent of anticipated contact was incompatible with the purpose and consequences of an adoption order.

Given judicial unwillingness to direct adoptive parents to maintain contact, birth parents and other relatives who anticipate contact and are subsequently disappointed have no option but to apply for leave to make an application under section 8 of the Children Act. Section 10(9) of the Children Act directs the court to consider certain matters when deciding whether to grant leave when the applicant is not the child concerned. The court must have regard to the nature of the proposed application for a section 8 order, the applicant's connection with the child and any risk that an application may disrupt the child's life to such an extent that he or she will be harmed by it. Within this legislative framework courts have been very cautious about granting leave. In *Re E (Adopted Child: Contact: Leave)* [1995] 1 FLR 57, the child concerned was placed for adoption by the local authority and her social worker promised the birth parents that photographs would be sent to them at intervals after adoption. Three years later the birth parents had not received any photographs of their daughter and they applied for leave to make an application under section 8 of the Children Act for an order enforcing indirect contact. Thorpe J, giving judgment in the High Court, expressed sympathy for the birth parents. He noted, however, that the adopters had always been opposed to any form of contact and, unless there were exceptional circumstances, courts were not prepared to impose contact on resistant adoptive parents. Furthermore, he thought there was a 'measurable possibility' that an application for a section 8 order might be disruptive for the child and prove to be harmful. The outcome of this case contrasts with the judgment in *Re T (Adopted Children: Contact)* [1995] 2 FLR 792. Here, the adopters agreed to provide annual reports to the sister of two children at the time they were adopted. It appears the adoptive parents changed their minds about indirect contact and failed to provide any information. The children's sister applied for leave to make a section 8 application but was refused by the County Court. She appealed and the Court of Appeal granted leave for her to proceed with an application. The Court found that the adopters' change of mind constituted a change in circumstances from the time the adoption order was made and there was no evidence to suggest that disruption or harm would be caused by the sister's application. Importantly, Balcombe LJ made it clear that it was unacceptable for adopters to give an undertaking about contact and then to break it without providing an explanation. The adequacy of their reasons will contribute to a court's decision about whether to grant leave.

Giving judgment in *Re C (A Minor) (Adopted Child: Contact)* [1993] 2 FLR 431, Thorpe J referred to section 10(9) of the Children Act 1989 and rehearsed the requirements for a court to give a 'former parent' or other birth relative leave to proceed to an application. He noted the permanent and final nature of an adoption order such that any re-opening of litigation post-adoption should only be allowed if circumstances had changed fundamentally since the adoption order was made. *Re S (Contact: Application by Sibling)* [1998] 2 FLR 987 confirms judicial unwillingness to give leave for post-adoption contact applications. In this case two siblings had been adopted into separate families and the girl was showing increasing distress at the lack of contact with her brother. The brother's adoptive mother was totally opposed to any form of contact and said the threat of proceedings was undermining her ability to care for him. The sister's adoptive parents wanted to facilitate contact. Hearing the case in the High Court, Charles J refused to grant leave for a section 8 application. This was primarily because there had never been any agreement about contact, the sister's unforeseen distress did not constitute a change in circumstances and an application was likely to cause disruption and consequential harm to the brother. Further, any initiation of contact might result in other birth relatives discovering the boy's address. Millett LJ in *Re T (Adoption: Contact)*, discussed above, was acutely aware of the burden placed on birth relatives who were promised contact at the time of adoption and then had to apply for leave when adopters reneged on their agreement. He suggested they could bypass the necessity for leave under section 10 of the Children Act 1989 if, when an adoption order was made, it included a record of agreed contact and stated that the court did not find it necessary to make a contact order. Additionally, the court should make a note that birth relatives included in contact agreements had a 'liberty to apply' (that is, a right to apply without leave) for a section 8 order if adopters subsequently withdrew their undertaking.

While it is argued that courts do not take a sufficiently interventionist approach to securing and enforcing post-adoption contact, they are clearly aware that contact is important for some children. For example, in *Re B (Minors) (Care: Contact: Local Authority's Plans)* [1993] 1 FLR 543, the local authority applied for an order under section 34(4) of the Children Act 1989 allowing it to terminate contact between two children and their mother. The authority had identified prospective adopters for the children and wanted to effect a placement. However, in the eighteen months since the care order was made on the basis of an adoption plan, the children had experienced frequent and unsupervised contact with their mother, she had cared successfully for another baby and her parenting skills had improved. The court therefore refused to make an order allowing termination of contact and directed the local authority to assess the mother's ability to resume care of her children. *In Re E (A Minor) (Care Order: Contact)* [1994] 1 FLR 146, the local authority applied during care proceedings for an order authorising it to refuse contact between two children and their parents so it could pursue a plan for adoption. The County Court judge made the order and the guardian *ad litem* and parents appealed. In the Court of Appeal Sir Stephen Brown and his colleagues were satisfied that continuing direct contact with their parents was in the children's best interests. The court was not opposed to adoption but suggested the local authority should make more effort to find adopters who would facilitate post-adoption contact. Allowing the appeal, Sir Stephen Brown said:

In short, even when the s. 31 criteria are satisfied, contact may be of singular importance to the long-term welfare of the child: first, in giving the child the security of knowing that his parents love him and are interested in his welfare: secondly, by avoiding any damaging sense of loss to the child in seeing himself abandoned by his parents; thirdly, by enabling the child to commit himself to the substitute family with the seal of approval of the natural parents; and, fourthly by giving the child the necessary sense of family and personal identity. Contact, if maintained, is capable of reinforcing and increasing the chances of success of a permanent placement, whether on a long-term basis or by adoption.

(p. 154/5)

Similarly, in *Re G (Adoption: Contact)* [2002] EWCA Civ 761 heard on 20 May 2002, Lord Justice Ward in the Court of Appeal commented approvingly on the potential benefits of post-adoption contact:

Moreover, when one is looking at the benefits of contact, in a case like this the benefit is the benefit that comes from the children simply knowing who the natural parental figures are. It is to remove the sense of the ogre, as they reach adolescence and begin to search for their own identity, with the double crisis not only of adolescence itself but of coming to grips with the fact that they are adopted. That is why the current research is in favour of some contact in adoption.

(Paragraph 14, transcript provided by Smith Bernal Reporting. See also *Family Law*, 33: 9)

This case concerned a father's appeal against termination of his contact during care proceedings under section 34(4) of the Children Act 1989 where foster carers intended to make an application to adopt his children. Lord Justice Ward allowed the father's appeal and stated that the appropriate time to consider contact issues would be when the adoption application was heard. Interestingly, however, he noted that when contact came to be considered during an adoption hearing for these children the applicants' views about contact would be 'virtually determinative of the question' if an adoption order was made. Thus, while courts are prepared to frustrate a local authority's plan involving termination of contact, they are not prepared to interfere with the exercise of parental responsibility by adoptive parents or to encourage further litigation post-adoption. Current case law suggests that it will take exceptional circumstances for a court to impose contact on unwilling adopters and a significant change of circumstances for it to grant leave for a section 8 application when an adoption order has already been made.

## Conclusion: policy development and judicial restraint

As we have seen, policy development with regard to openness in adoption has largely been concerned with the rights of adopted people to non-identifying and identifying information about their birth families. In this context, the Hurst Committee's (1954) recommendation that adopted adults should have a right to identifying information about their birth parent(s) has been refined over the years into a complicated package of statutory requirements in the Adoption and Children Act 2002. While practitioners have increasingly been making arrangements for direct and indirect post-adoption contact, it has been argued that policy and law have failed to keep pace with changing practice (Lindley 1997; Adoption Law Reform Group 2000; Casey and Gibberd 2001). It seems to be the case that policy development has been cautious about promoting post-adoption contact, although National Adoption Standards and the Adoption and Children Act now require agencies and courts to think about it at certain points in the adoption process. However, we think arguments for radical change in policy and judicial thinking are, for two major reasons, largely misplaced. First, there are no sustainable grounds for expecting policy and law to follow changing practice if practice itself cannot point to solid evidence that continuing contact is in children's long-term best interests. As we demonstrated in Chapter 2, research evidence on this front remains contested. Second, judicial thinking reflects the nature and consequences of adoption as a final order that constructs new families. If advocates for contact want adoptive parents to have something less than full 'ownership' and control of their children, then adoption must lose its distinctive character. It may also lose some of those qualities that enable it to work – security, assured permanence, commitment, a mutual sense of belonging, adopters' sense of 'entitlement' to their children – in short, those qualities enjoyed by ordinary families and reflected in everyday parent–child relationships.

The case law discussed in this chapter indicates the importance of negotiating and agreeing contact arrangements before an adoption order is made (Department of Health 2000, 2001b). It also points to the importance of educating, preparing and supporting adopters so they are persuaded about the importance of contact and feel committed to facilitating ongoing arrangements (Kedward *et al.* 1999). If this work is completed effectively, adoptive parents will be less likely to renege on agreements once they have safely achieved an adoption order. In future, research may provide clearer information about the relationship between different arrangements for post-adoption contact and children's long-term well-being. However, decisions about contact will still require an assessment of adults' and children's particular characteristics, attitudes, experiences and feelings that may or may not contribute to beneficial outcomes for participants. All this suggests that decisions about contact, ensuring contact is mutually acceptable and establishing conditions for the maintenance of contact lie more appropriately with developing practice than with achieving major changes in policy and law. Others (Cullen 1994; Masson 2000a) have similarly argued that issues associated with negotiating and supporting contact arrangements are best managed in a social and practice context rather than in court. This approach seems to be the preferred policy position in the National Adoption Standards' (Department of Health 2001b) reference to links and contact, which we discussed earlier in this chapter. The following chapters will consider these issues in relation to our own research with adoptive parents, birth relatives and children having direct (face-to-face) post-adoption contact. We will discuss the conditions under which individuals experienced contact as beneficial and identify those factors that introduced conflict and discomfort. Our research also suggests that the particular character of adoption can act to facilitate rather than to frustrate arrangements for post-adoption contact.

## Summary

- The Hurst Committee first raised issues concerning access to information, particularly for adopted adults, in its report of 1954. Subsequently, following the Houghton Committee's recommendations in 1972, section 51 was introduced in the 1976 Adoption Act. Section 51 gave adopted adults, adopted after 26 November 1976, the right to gain information from birth records held by the Registrar General. Those adopted before 26 November 1976 had to be counselled before they could access birth-record information.
- The Adoption and Children Act 2002 contains provisions in sections 56 to 64, which govern arrangements for the disclosure of 'protected' and other information to adopted adults and children and other persons. The provision of counselling services for individuals making use of these sections is also included.
- Since the early 1990s policy concern about access to information has been supplemented by arguments that policy-makers and courts should be more proactive in promoting and enforcing post-adoption contact for children. The Adoption and Children Act 2002 requires courts to consider any arrangements or proposals for contact when they make a placement or adoption order.
- Courts were able to attach contact conditions to an adoption order under the 1976 Adoption Act and have been able, since implementation of the Children Act 1989, to make a section 8 order for contact alongside an adoption order. However, they have been unwilling to use these provisions. Where adopters agree to contact, courts avoid making what seems to be an unnecessary order (see section 1(5) of the Children Act), and where they oppose contact, courts consider it inappropriate to interfere with adoptive parents' exercise of their parental responsibility. Courts have also been cautious about granting birth-family members leave to apply for a section 8 order after adoption, unless there has been a fundamental change in relevant circumstances since the adoption order was made.
- Policy, legislation and case law all point to the importance of negotiating, agreeing and supporting contact arrangements before an adoption order is made and of providing responsive mediation services to children, adopters and birth families if arrangements break down.

# 4 The study

## Research issues, methods and sample characteristics

### The study in context

In preceding chapters we outlined issues and debates regarding developments in adoption policy and practice, the role of adoption for children 'looked after' by local authorities and the significance of identity and contact for children who are separated from their birth families. As indicated in Chapter 2, evidence from research on post-adoption contact is equivocal and contested. Similarly, in his overview of Department of Health-funded research on adoption, Parker (1999: 48) notes that many studies fail to adequately specify the type and frequency of contact and the relationship status of birth relatives who are involved. He critically comments 'if our understanding of the issues surrounding contact is to be sharpened, much more information is needed about exactly what it comprises'. The methodological confusion to which Parker refers makes it difficult to estimate the extent of different contact arrangements and to assess their particular impact on individual participants. It is thus arguable that adults and children who negotiate, manage and experience contact are engaged in playing out a 'social experiment' (Quinton *et al.* 1997: 411) whose long-term consequences remain largely unknown.

Our research was conducted between September 1997 and April 1999. Given that issues about post-adoption contact have largely attracted the attention of academics and researchers, we wanted to know how adoptive parents, birth-family members and adopted children felt about the debate that was going on around them. Our study was therefore designed to include a sample of adoptive and birth families where it had been agreed that direct (face-to-face) contact would continue after adoption. The specific aims of the research were as follows:

- To understand the significance of adoption for those people most closely affected by this form of legal arrangement.
- To identify the advantages and disadvantages of direct post-adoption contact from the perspectives of adoptive parents, adopted children and birth-family members having contact.
- To identify what kinds of factors influence the extent to which direct post-adoption contact is experienced as beneficial or otherwise for those most closely involved.

- To understand the impact of direct post-adoption contact on the lives of adoptive families, children and birth-family members.
- To learn lessons for policy and practice about circumstances that indicate direct post-adoption contact is likely to be beneficial for children and those that suggest direct contact should be avoided.

In Chapter 1 we discussed the confusion that surrounds references to openness and direct and indirect contact. Throughout this book we use 'direct contact' to mean face-to-face meetings and 'indirect contact' to indicate other arrangements for one- or two-way communication of information. Indirect contact usually involves letters and other written and photographic material where the adoption agency is used as a post box. However, we also include anything other than face-to-face meetings, for example telephone calls, under the broad heading of indirect contact.

## Ethical and methodological considerations

It is important to give some attention to the methodological and ethical issues, which we had to navigate while designing the study. Much of the research on social work intervention with children has tended to focus on adults' perspectives, viewing children as too cognitively immature, emotionally volatile and ethically problematic to provide reliable accounts of their own experiences and feelings. This approach, which gathers data about children rather than from them, reminds us of Butler-Sloss's (1988: 245) cautionary comment in the Cleveland Inquiry that 'the child is a person and not an object of concern'. Although more researchers in the field of adoption are now talking directly to children (see, for example, Fratter 1996; Thomas *et al.* 1999; Macaskill 2002), many studies continue to privilege the accounts of adults over those of children. However, the 1989 United Nations Convention on the Rights of the Child and the 1989 Children Act both identify the importance of enabling children to express their wishes and feelings and require social workers and courts to consider them when they are making decisions. Additionally, there is now an enormous and growing literature about children's rights and particularly their right to participate in decisions that affect their welfare (see, for example, Dalrymple and Hough 1995; John 1996; Freeman 1997; Smith 1997; Save the Children 2000).

Against this background we were particularly concerned to hear the views of children for whom direct post-adoption contact had been agreed. The methodological shift in research, which seeks to engage children as 'active participants', is now well documented (Butler and Williamson 1994; Hill *et al.* 1996; Morrow and Richards 1996; James and Prout 1997). It is arguable that ethical and methodological issues become more pressing when research involves direct conversations with children, particularly when they are (or have been) 'looked after' by the state. Thomas and O'Kane (1998a: 337) discuss the distinctive differences between research with adults and with children:

In part the difference is due to children's understanding and experience of the world being different from that of adults, and in part the different ways in which they communicate. Above all it is due to the different power relationships. For instance, consent is complicated by the fact that, for research to be done with children, both children and adults may be required to give their consent. Confidentiality is complicated by the fact that adults may expect to be told about the private lives and thoughts of children for whom they are responsible. Protection from abuse is complicated by the fact that children are less able to protect themselves than most adults, and by the fact that social institutions have special rules for the protection of children.

There is a growing body of literature about the ethics and practice of research with children (Alderson 1995; Morrow and Richards 1996; Hill 1997; Thomas and O'Kane 1998a; Christensen and James 2000; Lewis and Lindsay 2000; Masson 2000b). Good practice guidelines have also been developed. These include, for example, the National Children's Bureau Guidelines for Research (1993) and the Code of Practice for Research Involving Children from the Centre of the Child and Society, University of Glasgow (no date). Alderson (1995) identifies ten areas for particular attention when conducting research with children:

- The purpose of the research.
- Costs and anticipated benefits.
- Respecting privacy and confidentiality.
- Decisions about selection, inclusion and exclusion of children as research respondents.
- Decisions about funding.
- Review and revision of research aims and methods.
- Information for children, parents and other carers.
- Consent (who gives consent and how).
- Dissemination (reporting and using the findings).
- The impact of the research process on children.

Power emerges throughout the literature as a consistent theme and Morrow and Richards (1996: 98) identify this as the *major* ethical challenge when undertaking research with children. Thomas and O'Kane (1998b) similarly point to the unequal distribution of power between researchers and children. They additionally draw attention to the power imbalance between children and important adults in their lives, which can impede children's full participation in research. In their study 'Children and Decision-Making', Thomas and O'Kane (1998b) found that powerful adults significantly influenced their ability to gain access to children. These dimensions of the research process resonate with our own experience and during planning we were challenged by methodological issues that required careful consideration. Issues about which we were particularly mindful can be summarised as follows:

- How to gain access to potential respondents and how to negotiate with various gatekeepers, for example, adoptive parents and social workers. This was relevant in achieving access, not only to children but also to birth relatives with whom they were having direct contact.
- Ethical considerations, most notably how to gain the informed consent of children, establish boundaries of confidentiality and ensure their well-being during the study.
- Knowledge of children's cognitive and emotional development, including language use and attention span.
- The development of appropriate research tools and strategies to facilitate children's engagement with the researchers, to enhance trust and to empower children in the expression of their own views.
- The interpretation and analysis of data.

Interpreting data is an issue for all researchers and Mayall (1994) comments on the socially constructed nature of respondents' accounts, no matter what their ages. However, she considers the effect of differential power between children and adults to be most acute at the point of interpretation rather than at the stage of data collection. Mayall (1994: 11) says:

> However much one may involve children in considering data, the presentation of it is likely to require analysis and interpretation, at least for some purposes, which do demand different knowledge than that generally available to children, in order to explicate children's social status and structural positioning.

In a similar vein, Qvortrup (1987) discusses difficulties that are inherent in adults' attempts to interpret meanings, nuances, intentions and motivations embedded in children's accounts of their lives and experiences, and suggests that this constitutes a problem for the sociology of knowledge. However, we wanted children to tell us about something that only they could convey. That is, how *they* experienced and felt about adoption and contact. We were aware that we were asking children to focus on a particular aspect of their lives for a relatively brief period. Their responses may not therefore reflect how they feel at different times when they are concentrating on something else or simply getting on with the everyday business of being children in a family, with their friends or at school. This does not mean, however, that children's thoughts and feelings are not valid in themselves when expressed in a particular context. Like Thomas *et al.* (1999) we have not sought to interpret children's accounts. We have accepted and presented children's stories at 'face value' as being meaningful to them. The practical significance of these ethical and methodological issues, and their accommodation in our work, will be considered throughout this chapter.

## Gaining access to adopters, children and birth relatives after adoption

Four agencies, three local authorities and one voluntary adoption agency took part in the study. We wanted to obtain as large a sample as possible so we decided not to be prescriptive about children's ages or the length of time they had been placed with their adoptive families. We asked participating agencies to identify all adoptive families where arrangements had been agreed for continuing direct contact between one or more of their adopted children and any birth relatives. The resulting sample therefore includes a broad age range of children who had been in placement and adopted for varying lengths of time. Agencies sent adoptive families, meeting our criteria, a letter and information leaflet about the research with an invitation to participate. When adoptive parents agreed to take part, the agencies passed on their details to the researchers who then contacted them direct. The four agencies initially contacted eighty-two adoptive families of which seven said that they did not want to participate in the research. This does not, however, necessarily reflect the total number of families for which direct post-adoption contact had been agreed. It includes those where the agencies were still in touch and, very occasionally, excludes those where social workers thought it was inappropriate to intrude. Of the remaining seventy-five families, we were unable to include a further fourteen in the sample because they did not respond to our letters. The final sample comprised sixty-one adoptive families and their ninety-six adopted children. Unfortunately, we do not know how far non-respondents differed in any important respect from respondents, particularly with regard to their experience of adoption and contact.

The research was designed to include semi-structured interviews with adoptive parents, children and birth relatives who were all part of the same adoptive/birth-family kinship network so that we could compare their experiences of contact and explore any differences or tensions emerging through their respective accounts. We refer to these sets of interviews as 'triangles' because they include all three parties to the same adoption and contact arrangements. Having obtained the sample of adoptive parents we needed to identify children and birth relatives where direct post-adoption contact had been agreed. Given the diversity and complexity of many contact arrangements, this inevitably proved quite difficult and gaining access to participants was far more problematic than we had anticipated. Contact had been agreed with a range of birth relatives and children were meeting with different combinations of birth parents, grandparents, siblings, aunts and uncles. Some contact arrangements involved social workers but most relied on direct co-operation between adopters and birth relatives. In those situations where social workers were no longer involved, adoptive parents were the only source of information about the whereabouts of birth relatives. Siblings with contact arrangements were variously placed in other adoptive families, in residential or foster care, with birth relatives or at home with parents. Some siblings were older and living independently.

It was clear that we would need adoptive parents' permission before we could talk to their children or initiate contact with birth relatives. Where siblings were 'looked after' by local authorities or birth relatives were subject to professional intervention, we also needed to liaise with social workers to obtain the consent of potential respondents and to ensure the absence of factors that might contraindicate their participation in research of this nature. Where possible, we asked adoptive parents to make initial contact with birth relatives. If birth relatives responded positively, their details were passed on to the researchers who subsequently wrote to them with an information leaflet about the study. This process proved extremely time consuming and on many occasions birth relatives (and social workers) were contacted more than once. There were also instances where adoptive parents or social workers did not want to approach birth relatives, usually because the situation was difficult and they did not want to risk 'rocking the boat'. Where adopters were happy about their children participating in the research we were also concerned to ensure the children gave their informed consent. To this end we prepared an information leaflet for children which described the research and introduced the researchers in a child-friendly way. We asked adopters to give the leaflet to children who could then decide whether they wanted to be involved.

Butler and Williamson (1994) describe how gatekeepers can act to bar access in research with children. In our study gatekeepers, most notably social workers, also presented barriers to the participation of significant adults. As previously noted, we had hoped to include a majority of 'triangles' in our sample, in anticipation that they would provide a particularly rich source of data and allow us to compare individual experiences of shared contact arrangements. In some families, however, we could not interview children because they were too young, had severe learning difficulties or their adoptive parents refused their permission. In a very few cases the children did not want to talk to us. We also faced problems in making contact with birth relatives because of difficulties in obtaining social workers' co-operation, siblings changing placement and/or social workers and adult birth relatives moving house and/or not responding to an invitation to participate in the research. Very occasionally, initially agreed contact had been lost and nobody knew how to locate relevant birth relatives. Continuing mental-health problems, unstable living arrangements and more pressing priorities compounded the difficulty of engaging birth relatives after an adoption order had been made. Fratter (1996) also indicates the problems associated with trying to involve birth relatives in research of this kind. All these factors meant that we were only able to *complete* eleven triangles. Table 4.1 identifies the number of adoptive parents, adopted children and birth relatives arising from the sample of sixty-one adoptive families and, of these, the numbers we were unable to interview for various reasons. The majority of adoptive parents were married couples. However, there were four single mothers and one single father in the sample. Table 4.2 identifies the broad reasons for our inability to interview some members of adoption triangles. We have already discussed some of the reasons why we could not make contact with birth relatives from adoption triangles. Given these factors, we were thus able to interview different combinations of adoptive parents, children and birth relatives for the sixty-one families in our sample. Table 4.3 identifies the groupings of individuals (different members of adoption triangles) who were interviewed in the overall sample.

*Table 4.1* Total respondents in sample and numbers interviewed in each group

|  | A/M | A/F | A/C | B/M | B/F | B/GP | B/A/U | A/S | NA/S |
|---|---|---|---|---|---|---|---|---|---|
| Total sample | 60 | 57 | 96 | 21 | 6 | 32 | 8 | 9 | 41 |
| Interviewed | 60 | 50 | 51 | 6 | 2 | 18 | 5 | 0 | 11 |
| Not interviewed | 0 | 7 | 45 | 15 | 4 | 14 | 3 | 9 | 30 |

*Key*: A/M adoptive mothers; A/F adoptive fathers; A/C adopted children; B/M birth mothers; B/F birth fathers; B/GP birth grandparents; B/A/U birth aunts and uncles; A/S adopted siblings *not* included in our sample of adoptive families; NA/S non-adopted siblings.

*Table 4.2* Reasons for inability to interview potential respondents

| Potential respondents | | Reasons for non-response |
|---|---|---|
| Adoptive fathers | 7 | refused to be interviewed |
| Adopted children | 17 | too young |
| | 9 | children refused |
| | 4 | adopters refused |
| | 1 | placement recently disrupted |
| | 5 | children with severe learning difficulties |
| | 4 | not appropriate due to specific circumstances |
| | 5 | interviewed but tapes inaudible |
| Birth mothers | 1 | lost contact with adopters after adoption |
| | 2 | refused |
| | 9 | problems making contact |
| | 1 | birth mother died |
| | 2 | adopters asked us not to contact birth mothers |
| Birth fathers | 2 | problems making contact |
| | 2 | adopters asked us not to contact birth fathers |
| Birth grandparents | 4 | refused |
| | 4 | problems making contact |
| | 3 | adopters asked us not to contact grandparents |
| | 3 | in hospital, depressed or died |
| Aunts/uncles | 3 | problems making contact |
| Adopted siblings (not in our sample) | 2 | siblings' adoptive parents refused |
| | 2 | siblings refused |
| | 3 | problems making contact |
| | 2 | lost contact with sample children after adoption |
| Non-adopted siblings | 1 | lost contact with sample child after adoption |
| | 3 | inappropriate due to particular circumstances |
| | 6 | siblings or their carers refused |
| | 20 | problems making contact |

*Table 4.3* Adoptive families grouped according to individuals interviewed

| Sample of 61 families grouped according to those interviewed | Individuals interviewed in each group | | | | | | | |
| --- | --- | --- | --- | --- | --- | --- | --- | --- |
| | A/M | A/F | A/C | B/M | B/F | B/GP | B/A/U | SIBS |
| Adoptive parents, children and birth relatives (triangles) | 11 | 11 | 18 | 4 | 2 | 6 | 4 | 3 |
| Adoptive parents and birth relatives only | 10 | 9 | 0 | 2 | 0 | 12 | 1 | 8 |
| Adoptive parents and children only | 19 | 15 | 33 | 0 | 0 | 0 | 0 | 0 |
| Adoptive parents only | 20 | 15 | 0 | 0 | 0 | 0 | 0 | 0 |
| Total interviewed | 60 | 50 | 51 | 6 | 2 | 18 | 5 | 11 |

*Key*: A/M adoptive mothers; A/F adoptive fathers; A/C adopted children; B/M birth mothers; B/F birth fathers; B/GP birth grandparents; B/A/U birth aunts and uncles; SIBS siblings *not* included in our sample of adoptive families.

## Research instruments and data collection

There were two stages of data collection. The first involved asking adoption-agency social workers to provide basic background information about the children in our sample. The second stage consisted of interviewing adoptive parents, birth-family members having direct post-adoption contact and children wherever possible. We asked social workers from the four participating agencies for information about parental agreement to adoption and grounds for dispensing with their agreement when this occurred, reasons for adoption plans and arrangements for direct post-adoption contact. Further details were requested about children's dates of birth, legal status, ethnicity, moves between placements prior to adoption and dates of placement for adoption and adoption orders. Social workers obliged us by completing questionnaires for the vast majority of children in the sample.

Semi-structured interviews were conducted with adoptive parents and, with their permission, were taped and transcribed. We invited adopters' views on a range of topics including their reasons for adopting and their experience of the adoption process, their initial reactions to the idea of direct post-adoption contact, agency preparation and the extent to which they felt involved in negotiations about contact. We asked about any changes in contact arrangements, their feelings about birth relatives having contact and their perceptions of the advantages and disadvantages of contact for themselves, their children and birth relatives. Adoptive parents were interviewed separately to allow for the possibility that they might express different views. Married adopters, however, had remarkably similar perceptions and we only differentiate between their comments in forthcoming chapters when this is of significance for our discussion. The same approach was used for interviewing birth relatives and our questions reflected the topics about which we asked adoptive parents. We wanted to know how birth relatives felt about adoption, how far they were involved in discussions about post-adoption contact, how they felt about the adoptive parents and the perceived advantages and disadvantages of contact for themselves, the children and adopters. Our questions were essentially open-ended and we did not offer lists from which respondents could choose alternative answers. Respondents' accounts were likely, therefore, to reflect feelings, attitudes and explanations that were foremost in their minds and of greatest significance to them. The downside to this approach is that respondents may not think beyond their immediate answers if they are not prompted by other options that are presented for their consideration.

## Talking to the children

When deciding how to engage children in talking to us about our research interests we were guided by several issues identified earlier in this chapter. We were concerned with enabling children to tell us about their experience of direct contact in situations where they were dependent on powerful adults to arrange, manage and control contact meetings. There was a danger that children would consider it too risky to divulge their feelings about social workers, birth relatives and their adoptive parents and this raised issues of consent, confidentiality and trust. Additionally, ways of communicating with children had to be adapted to their cognitive and linguistic abilities. Morrow and Richards (1996) suggest that employing a variety of research techniques, which allow children to feel part of the research process, can ameliorate the effect of adults' power. Some children may feel comfortable with a traditional interview, while others may find relatively formal conversations threatening or confusing. Sometimes children are more communicative when researchers talk and interact with them in the context of everyday activities (Beresford 1997).

We were aware that children are not a homogeneous group. The children in our sample had varied histories and experiences and they differed in terms of their ages and their cognitive and emotional development. It was important to ensure that children understood what our research was about, to allow time for questions and clarification, to convey our interest in understanding their thoughts and feelings and to reassure them that our conversation was private unless they wanted to share it with someone else. We explained that social workers had to make decisions about contact between children and their birth relatives and that it would be helpful for them to know what children thought of their arrangements. When visiting children we went armed for any eventuality and we followed their lead. Most adopters and children were happy for our conversations to take place without adoptive parents being present. Children talked, showed us their life-story books, produced photographs taken during contact visits, drew pictures and sometimes used practical props like measuring jars and beads to illustrate relative quantities of love, happiness, sadness, anger and so on. As an additional aid we developed a series of 'clouds' which were designed to encourage children to express themselves through writing or drawing pictures. The clouds used ideas from the *Anti-Colouring Book* (Striker and Kimmel 1979) and contained incomplete statements such as 'I have contact with', 'seeing them makes me feel', 'when I have finished seeing them I feel', 'I worry about' and 'what I would like to happen when I'm older is'. Children were asked to complete the statements in whatever way they wanted. Of the ninety-six children in the sample, we were able to talk to fifty-one about their experiences of adoption and contact. Eight of these children did not complete the clouds but a further eight children, who declined an interview, used the clouds to convey their thoughts. We were thus able to gain information from a total of fifty-nine children. Most of the 'non-response' from children was due to their young age or severe learning difficulties.

## Children's characteristics and placements

In our sample, a total of ninety-six children were placed with sixty-one adoptive families. Forty-three children were boys and fifty-three were girls. Many children had 'special needs' in the sense that they required adoption placements with siblings, they had experienced neglect and/or abuse and they had moved between several placements before joining their adoptive families. Four children had Down's syndrome, three had serious physical disabilities and two had significant learning difficulties. The majority (92 per cent) of children were white British and the remaining 8 per cent were of mixed parentage. All the white children were placed in white families, as were three of the children of mixed parentage. The remaining five children of mixed parentage were placed in racially matched families. Thirty-nine children were placed singly, thirty-six in sibling groups of two and twenty-one in sibling groups of three. Twenty-one (22 per cent) children were adopted by families which had initially fostered them. Children had lived with their adoptive families for varying lengths of time. When we conducted the study, 58 per cent of the sample children had been living with their adoptive families for between three and five years, 18 per cent for between six and nine years and 7 per cent had been placed between eleven and fourteen years earlier. Only fourteen (15 per cent) children had been placed with their adoptive families for two years or less. In most cases, therefore, direct contact had been ongoing for three years or longer. The majority of children (68 per cent) were under five when they joined their adoptive families, reflecting national trends in the age of looked-after children who are placed for adoption (Performance and Innovation Unit 2000: 12; Department of Health 2000: 2; Ivaldi 2000: 34). Table 4.4 identifies children's ages when they were placed with their adoptive families and at the time of the research. Relatively few children went straight from birth parents to their adoptive families without intervening placements unless, fortuitously, their first foster carers became their adoptive parents. Table 4.5 identifies placements away from birth parents for the children in the sample prior to their placement with prospective adopters.

*Table 4.4* Ages of children at placement with the sample family and at the time of the research

| Age of children | On placement number | On placement % | At research number | At research % |
|---|---|---|---|---|
| Birth to under 2 years | 24 | 25 | 0 | 0 |
| 2 to 4 years | 41 | 43 | 8 | 8 |
| 5 to 7 years | 23 | 24 | 27 | 28 |
| 8 to 10 years | 5 | 5 | 34 | 35 |
| 11 to 13 years | 3 | 3 | 21 | 22 |
| 14 years and over | 0 | 0 | 6 | 6 |
| Total | 96 | 100 | 96 | 99 |

*Table 4.5* Number and types of placement prior to adoption placement

| Separate placements with foster carers | Number of children | Additional placements/explanation |
|---|---|---|
| 0 | 12 | These children were largely those placed with foster carers who subsequently became their adoptive parents but one child had an adoption disruption and one child had spent several separate periods with grandparents. |
| 1 | 34 | Of these children, 2 had also had one placement in residential care, 1 had experienced a disrupted adoption placement, 4 had spent one period with grandparents and 2 had spent two periods with grandparents. |
| 2 | 21 | Of these children, 3 had also had one placement in residential care, 1 had spent one placement in residential care and one period with grandparents, 3 had spent one period with grandparents and 1 had spent three separate periods with grandparents. |
| 3 | 7 | Of these children, 2 had also spent two separate periods with grandparents and one had spent several periods with grandparents. |
| 4 | 5 | One child had also spent a period in residential care |
| 5 | 4 | One child had also spent a period in residential care |
| 6 | 2 | |
| 7 | 2 | |
| 10 | 1 | |
| No information | 8 | |
| Total | 96 | |

## Children's legal and 'looked-after' status

Adoption plans were made for the majority of children in our sample because social workers concluded that their birth parents were unable or unwilling to provide safe and adequate parenting. Most of the children had experienced neglect, emotional abuse and/or physical abuse prior to becoming 'looked after' by the local authority. A small number had also been sexually abused. It is, therefore, unsurprising to find that sixty children were subject to care orders when they were placed for adoption. In a further twenty-one cases the local authority had obtained an order 'freeing' the children for adoption (section 18, 1976 Adoption Act). The Wardship jurisdiction was used for seven children in exceptionally difficult or unusual circumstances, for example where a mother lacked capacity because of severe intellectual impairment and, in one case, where the children's mother was dead and their father did not have parental responsibility. Only eight children were accommodated under section 20 of the Children Act 1989 prior to their placement for adoption.

## Birth parents' attitudes to adoption and post-adoption contact

One or both parents of only twenty-four (25 per cent) children in our sample were willing or able to agree to their adoption. At least one parent refused their agreement for a further twenty-four children and at least one parent of thirty-eight children actively contested the adoption application. One birth mother lacked the mental capacity to make a decision about adoption. Both parents of one child and two mothers of six children were dead at the time of the adoption application. We were unable to obtain this information for two children. If we consider the eighty-nine sample children about whom we have information and where parents required to give their agreement to adoption were alive and capable of doing so, only 27 per cent of adoption applications attracted parental agreement. In his survey of children adopted from 'care', Ivaldi (2000: 51) similarly found relatively few parents (29 per cent) who agreed to adoption for the 953 children about whom information was available. Although our study was designed to include children who had arrangements for *direct* post-adoption contact with birth relatives, we discovered that many of them also had indirect contact with other members of their birth families. Overall, plans were made for sixty-two (65 per cent) children in forty-two (69 per cent) families to continue direct or indirect contact with at least one birth parent, most usually their mothers. Research on openness and adoption conducted in the USA and New Zealand has largely related to children who were voluntarily relinquished at birth. Children's characteristics and parental attitudes to adoption are, therefore, very different from those identified in our sample. Table 4.6 indicates birth parents' willingness to agree to an adoption order where they expected direct or indirect contact to continue after adoption.

*Table 4.6* Birth parents' responses to adoption proceedings where direct or indirect post-adoption contact was agreed

| *Adoptive families where direct contact was arranged with at least one birth parent: 29 (48%) adoptive families and 42 (44%) children* | | | *Adoptive families where indirect contact was arranged with at least one birth parent: 13 (21%) adoptive families and 20 (21%) children* | | |
|---|---|---|---|---|---|
| Order contested | Consent refused | Adoption agreed | Order contested | Consent refused | Adoption agreed |
| 7 families | 6 families | 13 families | 6 families | 3 families | 3 families |
| In a further three families involving contact with birth fathers, the fathers' consent was not required but birth mothers in two cases contested adoption orders. | | | The birth mother in one case was unable to give her views due to mental incapacity. | | |

## Direct contact: variability, frequency and arrangements

Our study reveals a highly variable and complex range of contact arrangements. For some children, direct post-adoption contact was agreed with only one birth relative while others had arrangements to meet several members of their birth families both individually and collectively. Siblings were the birth relatives most likely to have direct contact with children in our sample families. Nineteen (20 per cent) children had contact arrangements with siblings who had been adopted by families within the sample. Of the 117 birth relatives who we identified with direct contact arrangements, fifty (43 per cent) were siblings who had been adopted by families outside our sample or, more usually, who remained 'looked after', had achieved independence as young adults or lived with their birth families. Birth relatives who were least likely to have direct contact were fathers (5 per cent) followed by aunts and uncles (7 per cent). In addition to direct contact, forty-three (45 per cent) children in twenty-eight families were having indirect contact with one or more birth relatives. Unlike arrangements for direct contact, birth parents were more likely than any other relatives to have indirect contact.

In addition to the variety and different combinations of birth relatives with whom direct contact was agreed, the frequency of contact also varied across the sample. When we conducted the study, the majority of birth mothers had contact two or three times a year, but three saw their children six times annually and in one case, where the child had previously been fostered by his adoptive parents, meetings were every month. Contact for birth fathers was usually two or three times a year. In one case, again for a child whose foster carers had subsequently adopted her, the father's visits were at least monthly. Exceptionally, one birth father had fortnightly meetings with his two children while they were placed with prospective adopters. Social services intended to keep his contact arrangements under review in the anticipation that some direct contact would continue after adoption. The children, however, resisted contact and expressed such distress that arrangements were terminated shortly before adoption orders were made. Grandparents' meetings with the children varied between once annually and every month, with the vast majority of arrangements falling between four and six times a year.

This summary information hides the extent to which, by the time of our research, trusting relationships had developed between many adoptive parents, children and birth relatives so that original contact arrangements had become more flexible and informal. A negotiated number of contacts a year had evolved into overnight and weekend visits, joint holidays, shared family celebrations and so on. For many families and children there was frequent telephone and letter contact between meetings. Although adopters did not always give their addresses to birth relatives, we could identify only ten adoptive families where communication was one-way. In these cases contact visits were either arranged through social services or adoptive parents approached birth relatives, who did not have reciprocal contact information for adoptive families. The complexity and nature of contact arrangements in our sample are broadly consistent with findings by Murch *et al.* (1993), Lowe *et al.* (1999) and other studies (Parker 1999). Table 4.7 summarises the distribution of birth relatives where direct contact was agreed with the ninety-six children and their adoptive families in our sample.

We have been careful in this chapter to refer to arrangements *that were agreed* for direct post-adoption contact and where it was anticipated that contact would continue for all the children and families in our sample. However, direct contact with birth mothers was terminated at adoption for six children in two adoptive

*Table 4.7* Distribution of birth relatives with direct contact arrangements

| Individual and groups of birth relatives for whom direct contact arrangements were agreed | Number of children | Number of families |
|---|---|---|
| Birth mothers only | 8 | 6 |
| Birth fathers only | 6 | 4 |
| Birth mother and father only | 1 | 1 |
| Birth mother and siblings only | 13 | 10 |
| Birth mother and grandparents only | 6 | 3 |
| Birth mother, grandparents and siblings only | 4 | 3 |
| Birth mother and aunt/uncle only | 1 | 1 |
| Birth father, paternal grandmother and aunt only | 3 | 1 |
| Grandparents only | 9 | 7 |
| Grandparents and siblings only | 8 | 4 |
| Grandparents and aunts only | 4 | 2 |
| Aunts and uncles only | 1 | 1 |
| Siblings only | 32 | 21 |
| Total | 96 | 64 (unrelated children in three families had different contact arrangements) |

families because its continuation was not considered to be in the children's best interests. This also happened for two children who were having direct contact with their birth father. Over time, a further three children in separate adoptive families lost direct contact with their birth mothers. We will explore these losses in greater detail in Chapters 6 and 8. Additionally, we included two families in the sample where direct contact was continuing between adoptive parents and, in one case, a birth father and, in the other, a birth mother. Although the children were not included in contact, their adoptive parents hoped they could 'keep the door open' for future meetings when the children were older.

## Conclusion: trials, tribulations and rewards

It was something of a challenge to organise the data from our sample of adoptive families and the sub-samples of children and birth relatives with whom we were able to discuss adoption and contact. Difficulties arose because, although we were able to interview one or usually both adoptive parents in the sixty-one families, we were not able to interview all their children or all the birth relatives for whom direct contact had been agreed. In Chapter 6 we discuss the perceptions of adoptive parents from the sixty-one sample families. Chapter 7 considers information from forty-two birth relatives who were having contact with children in the sample families and who agreed to talk to us. In Chapter 8 we consider information from fifty-nine children about their attitudes and feelings in relation to adoption and contact. In this chapter we also take a more detailed look at sibling contact and discuss the views of eleven birth siblings who had contact with children in the study sample. The focus in Chapter 9 is on triangular relationships in eleven kinship networks where we were able to talk to adoptive parents, children and birth relatives who shared contact arrangements. Research respondents in Chapter 9 are thus brought together for the purpose of comparing their attitudes to adoption and contact. They constitute a sub-sample of adoptive parents, children and birth relatives whose views and feelings we have discussed separately in previous chapters.

When we were designing and conducting this research we sometimes wished we had chosen to survey people's attitudes to shopping or to ask children about their hobbies. Instead we had embarked on a study that concentrated on ethically, personally and socially sensitive issues – those associated with adoption and direct post-adoption contact. We were going to talk to children who had 'lost' their birth families and started a new future with strangers, to birth relatives who had 'lost' their legal status and to adoptive parents who had agreed to share their children with people from a frequently hurtful and traumatic past. We hope this chapter has conveyed something of the challenges as well as rewards that were involved in this undertaking and has introduced the complex contact arrangements with which we were confronted. In subsequent chapters we discuss relevant issues in detail, describe how adopters, children and birth relatives experienced direct contact and indicate factors that contributed to beneficial and problematic contact arrangements. All the names of our respondents have been changed to protect their anonymity.

## Summary

- The study sample, from three statutory and one voluntary agency, comprised sixty-one adoptive families and their ninety-six adopted children where arrangements had been agreed for direct (face-to-face) post-adoption contact.
- Interviews were conducted with sixty adoptive mothers, fifty adoptive fathers, six birth mothers, two birth fathers, eighteen birth grandparents, five birth aunts and an uncle, and eleven siblings who were either looked after by local authorities or living independently.
- We were able to talk to fifty-one adopted children about their experience of direct post-adoption contact and obtained information from eight others via completion of the 'clouds'. The children had lived with their adoptive families for varying lengths of time but 83 per cent of them had been placed for at least three years. Eighty-five per cent of children were aged between 5 and 13 at the time of the study.
- Arrangements for direct post-adoption contact were enormously varied. They involved different individuals and combinations of birth relatives, a variety of venues and a range of frequencies for contact visits.
- The vast majority of children in the study had been subject to statutory intervention because of neglect and/or physical and emotional abuse. Only eight children were accommodated by the local authority prior to their placement for adoption. Where parents were required to give their agreement to adoption and were able to do so, only 27 per cent of adoption applications attracted parental agreement. Overall, arrangements were made for direct or indirect post-adoption contact with at least one birth parent for 65 per cent of children in the sample.
- Birth siblings were most likely and birth fathers least likely to have direct contact arrangements following adoption. In addition to direct contact, forty-three children (45 per cent) also had indirect post-adoption contact with other members of their birth families.

# 5 Preparation and planning for direct contact

## Agencies, professional practice and contact

While there is a general international trend towards more open adoption, there is considerable variation between agencies in the extent to which they are prepared to support different forms of contact arrangements (Fratter *et al.* 1991; Grotevant and McRoy 1998; Henney *et al.* 1998; Neil 2002a). Clearly, agencies have a pivotal role to play in this context and professional practitioners' attitudes and beliefs will have a significant influence on contact planning. Given the incomplete and some-times confusing information from available research, it is perhaps not surprising that practitioners vary in their approach to the value of direct post-adoption contact and worry about its appropriateness in individual cases (Murch *et al.* 1993: 218). Silverstein and Kaplan Roszia (1999: 649) emphasise the importance of educating adoption professionals so they can achieve successful open adoptions. They assert that 'the entire agency system must embrace the belief that contact with birth families and others over time benefits all those touched by adoption'. Parker (1999) highlights the importance of early planning for direct contact and the need to integrate planning with the assessment and preparation of prospective adopters. Similarly, Jones (2002) identifies preparation as vital to helping prospective adopters understand the reality of adoption and long-term, well-resourced post-adoption support in contributing to effective contact arrangements.

The process of assessment can be an anxiety-provoking time for prospective adopters who may feel powerless and worried about saying and doing the right thing (Lowe *et al.* 1999; Bell and Cranshaw 2000). During this time practitioners are in a powerful position and can play an important role in helping prospective adopters to understand the additional challenges that come with adoption and in anticipating and responding to their anxieties or misapprehensions. Practitioners' values and attitudes can significantly influence the views of prospective adopters (Grotevant and McRoy 1998). A combination of positive attitudes towards birth families, education and the provision of emotional support is more likely to encourage prospective adopters to think about contact as being potentially beneficial for themselves and their children (Baumann 1999; Silverstein and Kaplan Roszia 1999). Neil's study (2002a) in the UK also confirms how adoptive parents' attitudes can be influenced by the formal and informal messages they receive from professional practitioners. She examined agency practice along the spectrum of contact arrangements and found that, while some form of post-adoption contact was planned for most of the 168 children in her study, direct contact was only anticipated for 17 per cent of children. Neil identified agencies' ambivalence and uncertainty even where plans for direct contact were already in place. This ambivalence does not help adoptive parents to feel confident about practitioners' decisions or to accept that contact is a good idea. Additionally, both Neil's work and Berry *et al.*'s study in the USA found that, where adopters felt pushed into agreeing with contact arrangements, they were less likely to succeed in maintaining contact or to experience it as beneficial (Berry *et al.* 1998; Neil 2000).

In this chapter we discuss how the adoptive parents in our study remembered their pre-placement preparation for contact and the process through which subsequent arrangements for contact were established. We asked adoptive parents at what point in their work with the agency they had been introduced to the idea of contact and what kind of preparation they had received. Our interest was focused on how far adopters experienced their preparation as helpful and whether, as a consequence, they felt adequately prepared for direct contact. By the time of our study, adopters were also able to evaluate preparatory work in the light of subsequent events. We were also interested in the process of planning for contact, how adoptive parents recalled the plan's introduction and the extent to which they had been involved in decisions about contact arrangements.

## Preparation for direct contact

Adoptive parents in our sample came from a variety of backgrounds, as we will explain in Chapter 6. Some already had children, some experienced infertility problems in extending their families and many were childless couples with little first-hand knowledge of parenting or adoption. In some cases they knew other people who had adopted and they had heard about open adoption. For many others, however, the idea of open adoption was something completely new. One adoptive mother illustrates the responses of many adopters when she recalled 'we were a bit shocked at first and we thought well, that's a bit modern'. Adopters from nineteen families in our sample had been experienced foster carers before adopting their children and had participated in preparation groups, which focused on the role of foster care. Facilitating contact with birth families was thus thoroughly covered with them in relation to fostering although, as we shall see later, becoming adoptive parents brought with it a whole raft of new feelings and expectations. With the exception of one adoptive couple, initially approved for inter-country adoption, all adoptive parents in the study had undergone training and preparation prior to agency approval. The majority of adopters were introduced to the idea of continuing contact at this stage and agencies conveyed the message that they should expect their children to have some form of post-adoption contact. Adoptive parents from thirteen families said they had not received specific preparation for contact, although most of them were approved many years ago and before contact became a significant issue. Adopters remarked:

The preparation was very much in general. The phrase 'open adoption', that was the new thing they were taking on. We had preparation groups for five to eight year olds and the chances were that all of us in the group were going to have an open adoption, so these words were used all the time.

Open adoption, you're told about all that and when you go and start saying you want anything other than a baby anyway, you go through all this because you know that the child is going to come with its own little parcel and its own family and all that entails.

Adopters described contact with birth families as one of the many themes included in their general preparation for adoption. On the whole, they were positive about the overall quality of the preparation they received. It was clear from their responses, however, that there was considerable variation between agencies in the quality of work that specifically addressed contact. Helpful preparation included the opportunity to meet adopters who had first-hand experience of contact and discussions with adopted people who shared their stories of a life without contact. Adopters found it useful to hear about relevant research and some adoptive parents had seen informative videos from New Zealand. Meeting birth relatives was considered particularly helpful. Many adopters described how this experience had transformed their attitude towards birth families and had helped them to understand their situations and feelings from a more sympathetic perspective. For example:

We did have one occasion where we actually had some birth mothers come in and talk to us about how they felt and it makes you feel really humble and you feel very sorry for them. You're certainly made aware through the training of what it must be like for those people. I don't feel any animosity towards them or anything like that.

Studies have demonstrated that contact cannot be achieved simply by emphasising children's needs or insisting that adoptive parents should comply with contact plans as a condition of approval and placement (Kedward *et al.* 1999; Neil 2002a and 2002b). In order for adoptive parents to feel comfortable about contact they need help to understand why contact is now included in most adoptions and why it is likely to be beneficial for themselves and their children. They also need to appreciate the purpose of particular contact arrangements in relation to children's experiences and relationships with members of their birth families. Additionally, prospective adopters should be encouraged to express their concerns and worries so these do not become future obstacles to facilitating contact or sources of resentment and suspicion. Responses from adoptive parents in our sample, however, suggest that these areas were not consistently covered and agency preparation was sometimes viewed as inadequate for helping them to cope with the realities of direct contact. Preparation tended to concentrate exclusively on children's needs for contact and insufficient attention was directed at helping adopters to anticipate their own feelings towards birth families and their responses to the kinds of management issues that might arise after adoption. For example, adopters said:

> We were well prepared for the mechanics of it, but how it affects you emotionally and how it affects your relationships with the children is something that isn't very well covered.

> There was no preparation as such, they stressed it was important for the child but there was no preparation about how to manage it, it was just 'see how it goes'.

Some adoptive parents described preparation groups that had been unhelpful. These were characterised by horror stories about difficult contact arrangements and had only served to alarm them. Some had been told of instances where prospective adopters had been rejected because they would not agree to contact. These adoptive parents had felt unable to voice their anxieties and uncertainty about contact in case this jeopardised their approval:

> We were sort of prepared. You go to groups and they tell you the most horrendous stories about what can happen during contact and we were a bit dubious.

> We were told basically in a nutshell, that if you didn't go for contact there would be less chance of you getting a child. You will say anything and do anything at that stage.

## Adoptive parents' attitudes towards contact

Agencies in the study were clearly getting the message across to prospective adopters that contact was important for children's well-being. The majority of adoptive parents said that, by the end of their preparation and approval, they had become convinced children should maintain some kind of contact with their birth families. However, although agencies seemed to have won over their minds, their hearts were another matter and many adopters said they had mixed feelings about contact at that time. Some adopters felt the agency had pressurised them into agreeing to contact and they thought it was a condition of their approval. These adopters acknowledged the importance of contact 'in theory', but remained emotionally ambivalent. They felt they had been given no choice if they wanted a child to be placed with them. Some adopters commented:

> Intellectually it gave us the idea that it was a positive thing to do but emotionally I think we would rather say that they're ours and forget about their past, but intellectually you realise that you can't do that. We felt a bit threatened but it was OK once we met their mum.

Yes we were nervous, if we'd had a choice I would still have gone for no contact. There was a lot of pressure to have to accept it because it was very much sold as this is what happens these days, if you want to adopt a child you've got to accept open adoption.

I felt we were obliged to do it. It was the new modern way of thinking. I was caught in a trap that social workers know best. I was open to anything then. We were desperate, we wanted to go through the process and take on board everything they were saying, we thought they were the experts so let's go for it because they know best.

I didn't like the idea of contact but it's one of those things you dare not speak about in case it affects your approval, you keep it covered up.

Other adopters reported that they felt positive about the prospect of contact. They were expressing an openness of attitude which Fratter (1996) identifies as important for successful contact arrangements. These adoptive parents said they had accepted the likelihood that any child placed with them would come with a contact plan and they were open and willing to work with it:

At group sessions there was a lot of force for contact and I don't think you could actually be opposed to something until you've tried it, so it was a case of suck it and see.

Yes, we had quite a lot of discussion about contact in preparation groups because most people start out believing that it's completely wrong and usually by the end of the groups and certainly by the time you've filled in the Form F, then you've begun to realise that it's important for the kids.

I don't think we needed persuading, I just think that you have to understand that this child has a background and it's accepting that and understanding what that, how that could impact with you really. In some cases there may not be any, in some cases there may be.

Macaskill (2002) found that while preparation played some part in shaping attitudes to contact, it was only minimally influential compared to the personal life experiences of adoptive parents. Most adopters in our sample accepted, intellectually at least, the importance of contact, but those who felt most comfortable about it at the point of placement were able to identify with some aspect of birth relatives' experience. One adoptive couple had just become grandparents themselves and could appreciate how hard it would be for their child's grandparents not to see her:

I felt sort of protective. We said, well what would happen, how would we feel if Ruth were our grandchild and we would be very upset and yes we acknowledged that they would be very upset that Ruth was no longer going to be in their family and readily accessible.

Another adoptive mother had been a step-parent and understood the need for some children to maintain contact with their birth mothers:

> I was fine about it, because remember I had been a step-parent which meant I was used to having a relationship with the children who were in my care and with their mother

The nineteen adoptive parents who had been foster carers prior to adopting were experienced in working with birth parents and they had developed an understanding of birth families' difficulties and the reasons for children's admission to care. Many had been involved with birth relatives who they described as challenging, threatening and demanding and were therefore less perturbed than other adopters by dramatic stories that often surround contact. For example, an adoptive mother who had previously fostered her child, had this to say:

> She'd [birth mother] turn up at my house drunk. She phoned any time day or night using unacceptable language, threatening to knife me or break the windows. Eventually it felt like we were adopting both of them, Felicity, and her mother as extra baggage. I tended to treat her mum as my own daughter.

All the adopters who had initially acted as foster carers said they had been comfortable with the idea of ongoing contact when the agency was considering their wish to adopt. However, adoption generated sometimes new and unexpected feelings towards their children and, post-adoption, some former foster carers became less comfortable with direct contact. Our findings suggest that factors which enable prospective adopters to feel some link with birth families are likely to be influential in shaping their attitudes to direct contact. Such factors include adopters' life experience, their role as foster carers and learning opportunities provided as part of their preparation to adopt. Other researchers have identified a relationship between adopters' ability to empathise with birth relatives and the continuation of mutually beneficial contact (Grotevant and McRoy 1998; Macaskill 2002; Neil 2002a).

During preparation, agencies introduce prospective adopters to different possibilities for openness, from sharing information one or both ways (indirect contact) to direct contact. At this stage, prospective adopters have little idea about the contact arrangements they may ultimately have to consider. Agencies can prepare adopters for the likelihood of contact, but it is not until the point of matching that they must confront the implications of real children, birth families and contact plans. Adopters may be sympathetic to the idea of contact but their willingness to accept it post-adoption may be eroded by their fears about its practical and emotional impact on their family life and relationships with their children (Parker 1999). Lowe *et al.* (1999) concluded from their study that adoptive parents generally favoured indirect contact. However, adopters were less concerned about the idea of direct contact than they were about the difficulties, which they anticipated would be thrown up by the 'dynamics' of meetings. At this early stage, adopters in our sample reported that their attitudes to contact were influenced by factors such as the type and frequency of contact, members of birth families who would be involved, birth relatives' feelings about adoption and birth relatives' histories of harming or protecting the children. They felt differently about contact with particular relatives, reflecting the work of Thoburn *et al.* (2000) who found a greater willingness to accept direct contact with siblings or other relatives than with birth parents. Preparatory work with prospective adopters is vital but agencies' responsibilities must extend beyond persuasion about the benefits of contact. A recurring theme in this book is the way in which adopters and birth families were left to grapple with issues arising from direct contact once the agency had negotiated and set up arrangements. One adoptive father understood the importance of contact and had agreed that his son should see his grandparents three times a year. Difficulties arose because of the grandparents' attitudes and behaviour and the adopters came to revise their original support for contact:

> That was a condition that came with it, which although you go through this six-week course, nothing and no-one can express what it's like. You know, they can never put it across. No way was I prepared for it. If they'd told me what it was like I wouldn't have gone through with it. We won't go through another one now.

## Meeting birth relatives involved in direct contact

Agencies frequently arranged meetings between birth relatives and prospective adopters prior to placement. While some adoptive parents remembered feeling more sympathetic towards birth relatives after preparation groups, they nonetheless described their nervousness, anxiety and apprehensive about meeting them. The meetings were always highly significant and emotionally charged and many adopters explained that their initial fears dissipated when they were able to talk to birth relatives and to see them as real people. One adoptive mother recounted agreeing to direct contact for her two daughters with their older brother who was fostered. It was suspected that the children's brother had been involved in a sexually abusive relationship with them and the adopters were anxious about continuing contact. However, their fears were allayed at a preliminary meeting:

> We were asked to meet the girls' mother, which we agreed to. At the time we agreed to meet the girls' brother in his foster home. We were both very nervous about this. We had the meeting with their mother, cleared up a few cobwebs and then had the meeting with their brother. We really liked him, so were quite happy about contact. Meeting him settled any reservations we had.

Social workers have an important role in supporting prospective adopters when they meet birth relatives for the first time and their attitudes can be influential in both positive and negative ways. Some adoptive parents in our study were involved in meetings with birth relatives who were opposed to adoption and in these instances relationships between birth relatives and social workers were often problematic. Adoptive parents, however, were sometimes able to engage with birth relatives in ways that were helpful. They could discuss their concern about the children's well-being and talk about possibilities for contact. Fratter (1996) and Macaskill (2002) also found that introductory meetings could be constructive even when birth relatives were hostile about adoption plans. The adoptive parents of three siblings in our sample recalled their concern about contact arrangements with grandparents and their anxiety about meeting them. They were particularly worried because the grandparents were opposed to adoption and had an acrimonious relationship with the children's social worker. The social worker did not agree with the plan for contact, which had been proposed by the guardian *ad litem*. However, when the adopters met the grandparents they were able to see them as ordinary people who were genuinely concerned about their grandchildren:

> Before we met them it was quite daunting because she [social worker] had built up this kind of ogre, so we were quite panicked to be honest. What are they going to think of us and what effect is it going to have on the children and it's quite daunting going into that situation. But after the first meeting we were quite relieved when we came out not having met the ogre that we thought we were going to and having found them quite nice and I think they were relieved because they didn't want them taken away. They had tried to look after them and failed and so had all that to live up to and I think when they met us it was a relief to them.

Some adopters, however, had found meetings with neglectful or abusive birth parents particularly difficult:

> It came home to me that these people were cruel to my children.

> When you get to the stage of meeting their birth parents, seeing their attitude, it makes it very difficult to look them in the eye.

## Planning for contact

Parker (1999) suggests that the implications of various kinds of contact should be clarified with prospective adopters and that adoption panels should consider contact proposals alongside their assessment of adoption plans. Information should include specific details about arrangements for contact and a statement of intention is not enough. The adoptive parents in our sample felt they had emerged from working with the agency with an expectation that some form of contact would be required for their children. They were aware, nonetheless, that they could exercise some choice about accepting particular children and could negotiate the type of contact they felt able to live with. It was clear from their responses, however, that when they were presented with a possible placement, contact plans were incorporated as 'part of the package'. This hindered their willingness and ability to hesitate or to object to contact since they risked having to wait for an alternative match:

> To a degree, yes, we had a choice. If we were offered a child and contact was involved and we didn't want that, we'd have to consider another child, we couldn't consider this one.

> No, not really, there was no choice. Well the way it was worded, I knew there would be some form of contact and that would be part of the deal. We didn't have an option. If we'd said no, then I don't think we'd have got him.

Adopters were largely presented with information about children for whom contact planning was already under way, although detailed arrangements had not always been resolved. All the children who were placed with our adopters had been looked after and most had experienced sustained and regular contact with their birth families. The change from rehabilitation to adoption planning required a revision of contact arrangements and sometimes the anticipated nature and frequency of contact remained uncertain when children were placed for adoption. In some situations, adopters had remained unable to consider specific contact details and had accepted their children knowing that plans remained unclear. Contested and protracted adoption proceedings and conflict between social workers, birth parents, guardians *ad litem* (now children's guardians) and lawyers left prospective adopters feeling excluded and uncertain about the kind of contact that might come with adoption. We wanted to know how far adopters felt they had been involved in the process of planning detailed contact arrangements. Their responses fell into four categories. First, agencies proposed a plan for contact, which had formed the basis for negotiation with adopters about detailed arrangements. Second, agencies had already worked out a detailed plan, which left no room for negotiation or adjustment, although adopters had felt able to accept this. Third, those cases where adopters had been excluded from detailed planning and remained upset and unhappy about contact arrangements. Lastly, some adopters said they had pushed the agency into supporting contact and working out a plan. Table 5.1 summarises how adopters described their experience of contact planning.

## Contact planning was agency led: adopters agreed with the plan and felt involved

In forty-five families (74 per cent), adopters reported that the agency had proposed a plan for contact with which they were prepared to agree. Their experiences differed, however, in the extent to which they were involved in discussing detailed arrangements. Adoptive parents in thirty-three families felt they had been allowed to participate fully. They were presented with the agency's intention that direct contact should continue, but were invited to discuss and agree decisions about

*Table 5.1* Managing early contact planning

| Decisions about contact plans | Number of adoptive families | % |
|---|---|---|
| Planning was agency led: adopters agreed with the plan and felt involved | 33 | 54 |
| Planning was agency led: adopters agreed with the plan although they were not involved | 12 | 20 |
| Planning was led by the agency/court/guardian *ad litem*/lawyers: adopters accepted the plan but remained hostile to its implementation | 10 | 16 |
| Planning was initiated by the adopters | 6 | 10 |
| Total | 61 | 100 |

frequency, location, supervision and ways of arranging meetings. In eighteen families, adopters had also been involved in negotiations with guardians *ad litem* and birth relatives' solicitors. Adopters recalled:

> It was an open discussion when contact was set up. They said there was contact, but how we were going to work it, that was fully discussed.

> We had meetings with everybody's social worker, we all got together and decided how contact was going to be worked out. We had quite a big say in what went on. There were issues we brought up they hadn't thought about. We were totally involved right from the start to finish. To a certain extent we had quite a lot of say in what went on.

> There was actually a choice in that sense about how much or how little.

Adoptive parents in fifteen families were left to negotiate the details of contact arrangements, with little or no professional help. The majority of these cases involved contact with siblings who were living with other adoptive families and the adoptive parents reached a mutual agreement about the frequency and venue for contact. In other kinship networks adopters and birth relatives met and managed to negotiate mutually acceptable arrangements. While most adopters said they had been happy about how contact arrangements were agreed, social workers should be aware that prospective adopters and adoptive parents might need their help. One adoptive mother found it difficult to establish arrangements and would have preferred some professional support:

> It was very much up to us to arrange everything, which is where the problems were really, because we were doing a lot of chasing around and ringing up. At the time I felt OK about it, but as soon as I realised that it wasn't going to be that easy to set up all the time I think it would have been better if somebody else had set it up and managed it.

Adopters valued having been involved in negotiations about detailed arrangements for direct contact. They felt that the views of all parties were taken into consideration and that this enabled everyone to accept and to be clear about contact arrangements from the beginning.

## Contact planning was agency led: adopters agreed with the plan although they were not involved

Adoptive parents in twelve families had been presented with a plan for contact but were not involved in negotiating detailed arrangements. In these cases, the details had already been decided, their views were not invited and they had to choose whether to accept the plan for contact as it was presented to them. Most of these situations involved children who had been in foster or residential care and contact arrangements with birth relatives were already well established. An expectation of continuing contact was thus premised on longstanding arrangements:

> It was always a factor right from the first interview. It was just accepted that we would carry it on because the children had been in the same home together and there was never a question of them not seeing each other.

> We were treated with respect but I don't think we had a contribution. We just said fair enough, we'll accept whatever's been happening. It seemed reasonable.

In these instances, adopters had generally been content to accept the plan for contact as arrangements were already in place and they could see that contact was working. In three cases, however, plans for contact had not been finalised before the children moved into their adoptive homes. Adopters in these situations had felt disadvantaged because they were not agreeing to functioning plans that were already tried and tested. These adopters expressed more ambivalence about contact, but felt they had little choice about whether to accept the plans. They said:

> It was put to us that it was important for the child so we accepted it. It was a necessary evil.

> We forced ourselves to accept it because they told us it was in her [the child's] best interest.

In all these situations, adopters had been particularly anxious about meeting birth relatives. Once contact was established, however, it continued to work satisfactorily and the adopters were happy for it to continue.

### Planning was initiated by the adopters

Adoptive parents in six families reported that they had pushed social workers to sort out plans for direct contact. In all but one of these families the adopters were experienced foster carers and had adopted their foster children. Three adopters were keen for their children to maintain contact with siblings who were adopted elsewhere. One adoptive couple had been in regular contact with their child's birth mother prior to adoption and had been working towards rehabilitation. When rehabilitation proved unsuccessful, they signalled their wish to adopt the child and the local authority terminated contact. The adopters were aware of the birth mother's distress and, in an effort to help her, they offered to see her once a year so she could maintain a link with her child and keep the door open for future meetings.

Adoptive parents of one child had previously provided respite care for him and had been in regular contact with his birth mother and grandmother. Because of his disability, social services did not think direct contact was necessary. However his adoptive parents thought that, as he had experienced frequent contact prior to adoption, this should continue. They discussed this with the guardian and birth mother's solicitor and contact arrangements were agreed:

> He saw his birth mother every two weeks and when we were thinking and talking around adoption, we felt it was probably good for him to have some form of contact and although it was not prescribed in the court judgement, we had no objection to contact. His mother was opposed to adoption and she only agreed if he came to us and we were happy for contact to continue.

Another adoptive family had a child with Down's syndrome. Her parents had relinquished her at birth. They did not want any form of contact, but her maternal and paternal grandparents wanted to see her. Her adoptive mother, a single parent, was estranged from her own parents and did not want her daughter to grow up feeling isolated from her extended family. To the surprise of social services, which considered direct contact to be unnecessary, the adoptive mother requested their help in arranging twice-yearly meetings with her daughter's maternal and paternal grandparents. While these adoptive parents were all very different, they shared a sense of openness about adoption and contact and felt sympathetic towards their children's birth families.

### Contact planning was led by the agency or other professionals: adopters accepted the plan but remained hostile to its implementation

The remaining ten situations involved contact planning that was either agency led, driven by recommendations from the child's guardian or promoted by arguments from birth relatives' solicitors. Adoptive parents had been unhappy with the plan for contact and, although they accepted it, they remained hostile to its implementation. In all these cases, adopters felt they had not been involved in the planning process and some had been forced into accepting a greater frequency of contact than they had originally anticipated. Adoptive parents from one family had agreed to twice-yearly contact, but at the last minute social services increased this to three meetings without consulting them. Another child's adoptive parents had accepted direct contact with his birth mother and siblings but were dismayed about their exclusion from detailed negotiations about how this would work:

> We were told it was three times a year, we were not involved. We didn't have a choice. We were disappointed. After putting yourself out to go along with the plan, then we didn't have a say in how much or how long. That was arranged by social services with our son's mother and then taken to court to be confirmed. I go along with it for his sake.

Sean's adoptive parents had been unhappy with the level of contact that was imposed on them. He had originally been placed with them for long-term fostering and had frequent contact with his birth mother, grandparents and siblings. Over four years later, they finally adopted him and, while they agreed that contact should continue, they anticipated a reduction in its frequency. However, the guardian *ad litem* took a different view and they were left with monthly contact, which they thought would be difficult to sustain in the long term. While, at the time of our research, these arrangements had continued for eight years, they had not been unproblematic. The adoptive father said:

> We were stitched up by the guardian – he made the recommendation to court. Both social services and ourselves were stitched up, but they didn't argue the case either. But that was that social worker, she was frightened to death.

In three cases, adoptive parents said they had been forced to accept the recommendations of the child's guardian. Sally is severely disabled and was placed with her adoptive parents at birth. Her adopters had stated in their assessment that they did not want a child placed with them for whom direct contact was the plan and the placement was made on this understanding. However, shortly before the adoption hearing the social worker had phoned to say the birth parents would not agree to adoption unless they could see Sally once a year. By this time, Sally had been placed with them for seven months and they were frightened of losing her if they rejected direct contact. Sally's adoptive mother said:

> We were emotionally blackmailed into it. I feel very resentful because of the way they did it. We have seen them three times now and it's a real blight on my life. In fact it's ruined my life.

Adoptive parents of two children had been faced with a similar situation. The children were in foster care for eleven months prior to being placed with their adoptive parents and a further eighteen months elapsed before the adoption hearing.

Throughout this time, the children had been seeing their birth parents. The birth parents actively contested adoption orders and, although social services did not consider contact to be in the children's best interests, the guardian disagreed. At some point during the adoption hearing the adopters said they had received a telephone call from the court asking them to agree to direct contact. They explained:

> We got a phone call at seven o'clock in the evening asking if we would agree to birth family contact and we had to decide before eight thirty. We were put in an emotional blackmail situation. The court made an order and it was emphasised that we had to adhere to it or face imprisonment. I felt it was totally ridiculous. It was a format reached by the guardian relating to the rights of the birth father which they wanted us to sign.

Our understanding of this situation is that the adopters thought an order would be made if they did not agree to direct contact. The adoptive parents were adamant that they would not force the children to see their birth father. With the help of their solicitor, and in negotiation with the birth father, they came to a compromise and agreed to meet the children's birth father once a year. The adopters promised to ask the children if they wanted to accompany them to these meetings. At the time of the research, the adopters continued to see the birth father without their children.

Parents in two adoptive families said they had been forced to accept a contact plan that was decided by social workers who did not consult them. In both cases, the guardian *ad litem* had intervened at the adoption hearing and the proposed plan for contact was revised. Adopters said:

> Social services had a plan, they wouldn't listen to us, they had a plan and they would stick to it. It was drummed into us that it was for the child's benefit so we just caved in.

These cases are two of the three in which contact with birth parents was terminated at adoption. Adopters in this group felt they had been let down by agencies and sometimes by the courts. It is perhaps unsurprising that, at the time of our research, adopters described most of these contact arrangements as problematic.

## Frequency of contact arrangements

Plans were made for three-quarters of the children in our sample to see their birth relatives between once and four times a year. Meetings of six to twelve times a year were less common. Fifteen children were seeing different relatives on different occasions, resulting in numerous contacts each year. For example, contact was agreed for one child with his birth mother three times a year, grandmother six times a year and siblings six times annually or more frequently. Table 5.2 summarises

*Table 5.2* Frequency of contact arrangements

| Frequency of contact | Number of children | % |
|---|---|---|
| 1–2 meetings per year | 27 | 28 |
| 3–4 meetings per year | 41 | 43 |
| 6 meetings per year | 6 | 6 |
| 12 meetings per year | 7 | 7 |
| Multiple contacts per year | 15 | 16 |

the frequency of contact arrangements. Because of the complexity of contact for children seeing more than one birth relative on different occasions, these are recorded as multiple contacts per year. Although post-adoption contact had been planned for three children in the category of one to two meetings per year, the children were never involved in contact meetings. Contact was terminated for one child at the adoption hearing but the adoptive parents agreed to meet their child's birth mother once a year. Two children resisted contact with their birth father, but their adoptive parents continued to see him once a year and were willing to take their children if they wanted to go.

## Agency involvement in post-adoption contact arrangements

With the exception of six families where adopters pushed for direct contact, all the contact arrangements were initiated by the agency, the guardian *ad litem* or birth relatives' solicitors. Post-adoption, social workers remained involved in contact arrangements for only a minority of children. At the time of the research they continued to play some role in contact for only eighteen children in the sample. Social workers had to remain involved with eight families because their contact arrangements included looked-after siblings. After an adoption order had been made, the majority of children depended on their adoptive parents and birth relatives to arrange contact. These contacts were less formal than those involving professionals and took place either at neutral recreational venues such as the zoo or McDonald's or at adoptive parents' and birth-family homes. Contacts controlled by social workers tended to be less frequent than meetings that were agreed between adopters and birth relatives. In some instances, social workers had recommended caution about how adopters should manage contact. Neil (2002a), in her study of agencies' contact planning, suggests that restrictive plans can convey negative messages to adopters about the safety and value of direct contact. One adoptive mother in our sample described how the social worker had advised them not to disclose their address and phone number to their child's birth mother:

> They were frightened of something happening that shouldn't and they told us not to give her our phone number. When we got to know her we decided to give it to her and she comes to our house now and everything has improved since then.

Many adopters commented that, while they appreciated the early assistance of professionals, they came to prefer direct communication with birth relatives as this enabled them to develop more relaxed and natural relationships. One adoptive father described his experience:

> Initially contact was handled by social services. Sean was collected from here by them and was taken to where the contact was. Eventually we took him and dropped him off in a children's home where his siblings were. From there he was collected by his grandparents and after a short while they would take him to the home and we would pick him up from there. It progressed from that to us meeting grandparents and handing Sean over to them and then returning later the same day to pick him up. Most of the fall-outs were caused by social services not passing messages on. They didn't like social services and there was always animosity between them and that caused a lot of the problems we had. Once we started taking over the contact meetings, 90 per cent of the problems just fell away.

Another adoptive mother said:

> And then I hated this idea of contact with social services and I didn't think it was good for the boys. Their birth mum was very frightened being near the social services building and someone was always bobbing their heads round the door saying 'is everything going alright?' So, we decided where can we go for all of these contacts and what can we do – just to get social services out of our hair so to speak and to make contact normal. So we hit on this place and the first time we did this we realised how different the contact was. It was just unbelievable – everybody was just so normal and relaxed. And their mum changed, changed completely because she no longer felt she had someone looking over her shoulder. It was lovely and that is what we have done ever since. And then two years into the contact, I decided I was sick to death of all these letters flying backwards and forwards through social services and the children's birthday cards and Christmas cards were all arriving late because they had to go through this system. So I gave her [birth mother] our phone number. Then a little while ago she came here and it was very nice and relaxed.

## Conclusion: agencies and planning for direct contact

As in other studies, our research highlights the significant role of agencies in preparing prospective adopters for contact and involving them in planning detailed arrangements. However, adopters' accounts suggest that agencies tended to concentrate on negotiating and agreeing contact arrangements without thinking about future developments and the need for ongoing support. Additionally, the advice and support that was provided in the early stages of contact often took the form of a rather 'blunt instrument' and failed to tailor arrangements in the light of adopters' and birth families' very specific needs. Negotiation, agreement and clarity in contact planning are important features of early work. However, agencies must acknowledge and prepare adopters and birth families for changes that may occur over time in response to the particular needs and circumstances of individuals (Grotevant and McRoy 1998; Logan 1999; Lowe *et al.* 1999; Neil 2000). By the time we conducted this research, contact arrangements for forty-eight children in our sample families had changed from the original agreements. The way in which agencies manage initial decisions about contact may provide adopters and birth families with a willingness and ability to continue working at their arrangements. Ongoing co-operation, communication and flexibility will enable participants in contact to re-negotiate their arrangements until they find a mutually acceptable 'comfort zone' in which they can work together (Grotevant and McRoy 1998: 174).

## Summary

- We asked adoptive parents in our sixty-one sample families whether they had felt adequately prepared for direct contact and to what extent they had been involved in planning and agreeing contact arrangements.
- Adopters in thirteen families could not recall any agency preparation that focused on contact. The remaining adopters said that contact had been a central feature of agencies' preparatory work with them. However, agencies concentrated on persuading prospective adopters that children needed contact and gave insufficient attention to anticipating the needs, feelings and management issues that might confront adopters, children and birth families over time.
- Most adoptive parents said the agencies had conveyed a clear expectation that they would have to accept some form of post-adoption contact for their children. Many adopters agreed that, in principle, contact was likely to benefit their children but some remained anxious about the emotional and practical implications of contact. They frequently felt unable to voice their worries in case this affected approval and subsequent placement.
- Agencies varied in the extent to which they had involved adopters in negotiating and agreeing contact plans. While all the adoptive parents in our sample had accepted contact plans at the point of placement, ten families felt they had been excluded from planning and had been forced to implement direct contact arrangements to which they were opposed. Adoptive parents in a further twelve families said they had been presented with contact plans which had been decided without their participation. In these cases, however, contact was already established and the adopters were happy that it appeared to be working. Some adopters had remained uncertain about contact arrangements until the adoption order was made as guardians *ad litem*, solicitors and courts intervened in social services planning.
- Preparatory work with prospective adopters is vital in developing their willingness and ability to accept and manage ongoing contact. However, agencies can do much more to facilitate successful contact arrangements. They should help adopters to anticipate issues that might arise over time and discuss ways of responding to these. Agencies can support prospective adopters and birth

families through initial meetings. All participants in contact arrangements should be included in discussing and agreeing detailed plans, and agencies should try to anticipate the likelihood of later intervention in planning. Social workers should avoid giving 'blanket' and overly controlling advice about the exchange of information and should give adopters the confidence to make their own informed decisions. Lastly, agencies should remember that contact arrangements may run into difficulties and pre-adoption contact planning is only the beginning of a long process.

# 6  Adoptive parents
## Perspectives on adoption and direct contact

## Adoptive parents and adoption

Howe (1996: 6) argues that the role of adoptive parents has become increasingly complex. He suggests that despite this, policy and practice developments in adoption have focused attention on children and their birth families to the virtual exclusion of any concern with adopters' experiences, feelings and insights. In order to redress the balance, Howe interviewed adoptive parents in 120 families whose adoptions had been finalised in the 1960s and 1970s. Savas and Treece (1998: 319) also think that 'the needs of adoptive families in general should be accorded greater recognition than is presently the case'. This line of argument does not intend to minimise the importance of children's and birth-families' needs, but acknowledges the significance of potentially different interests between the parties to adoption arrangements. As we have noted in preceding chapters, advocates of post-adoption contact tend to argue from the premise that contact is good for children and it is the social and legal nature of adoption and the expectations of adoptive parents that must change to accommodate contact. Put more bluntly, adoption, adopters and judicial attitudes combine to frustrate the arrangement of contact in the first instance or act to protect adoptive parents from any consequences if they break their promise after contact has been agreed. Happily, our study is able to consider the perspectives of participants approaching adoption from all three sides of the adoption triangle and this chapter concentrates on adoptive parents. It is not our intention to privilege one particular perspective over another. However, to understand the relationship between adoption and possibilities for continuing direct contact, it is vital that we should explore the expectations, feelings and views of adoptive parents. Our research only tackles one situation – where arrangements were agreed for adopted children to maintain direct post-adoption contact with birth relatives. Practitioners need to know more about the circumstances and attitudes of those adopters who are resistant to contact in order to develop approaches that effect and support change and maximise opportunities for contact when it is considered to be in a child's best interests. The adoptive parents in our sample have much to tell us about the conditions under which contact works well and is experienced as beneficial for themselves and their children. Additionally, our research leads us to the conclusion that adoption can, in appropriate circumstances, act to promote and sustain contact rather than to frustrate it.

We interviewed adoptive parents from sixty-one families where arrangements for direct post-adoption contact had been planned and agreed between the parties. As we noted in Chapter 4, 85 per cent of children had experienced direct contact for at least three years since placement with their adoptive parents. Arrangements were continuing for fifty-six families at the time of the research. Of the adoptive parents in our sample families, forty-two had been approved for adoption placements and nineteen had initially acted as foster carers for children who they subsequently adopted. In the latter case, by the time an adoption plan was finalised, foster carers had become attached to 'their' children and felt they had a good understanding of the children's needs. They were not about to let social services move the children to alternative adoption placements. Thirty (71 per cent) of the prospective adopters wanted to adopt because of infertility problems; two families already had adopted children and the remaining twenty-eight were childless. In the foster-carers' group, only two families were childless because of infertility. Ten prospective adopters already had birth children, as did fifteen of those initially acting as foster carers. However, of the ten prospective adopters six were motivated to adopt because of fertility difficulties in extending their families and only four chose to adopt for purely altruistic reasons. Three foster carers similarly experienced fertility problems in having more birth children. Two single adoptive mothers were approved for adoption and neither had birth children. Both single adoptive mothers who began as foster carers had one child each who was born to them. We think it is important to note the very small number of adoptive parents who were primarily motivated by an altruistic desire to accept children who needed a family. It might be thought that altruistic adopters would be more likely to facilitate direct post-adoption contact and that involuntarily childless couples would be less willing to 'share' their children with birth families. This is certainly not the case in our sample. Neither is it the case, as is sometimes suggested, that adoptive parents who begin as foster carers are more used to managing direct contact and more comfortable with it after adoption. Whether our families started out to foster or adopt, the children became unequivocally theirs following adoption and, in the vast majority of cases, they spoke about the rewards and trials and tribulations of family life much as any parent might do. Their attitudes to contact derived from much more complicated factors than their original motivation or prior experience as foster carers.

## Opposition to adoption: birth families and contact

Between them, the sample families had adopted ninety-six children. As we explained in Chapter 4, the majority of children were subject to care orders or other forms of statutory intervention because of a history of abuse and/or neglect, they were over a year old and many needed placements that could also accommodate their siblings. We also noted that adoption orders in respect of only 24 (25 per cent) children in the sample were made with parental agreement. Obtaining agreement from parents whose consent was required obscures the impact of several birth mothers who were only willing to agree at the final adoption hearing, having changed their minds or resisted adoption over many months of social-work planning and legal proceedings. Our point here is that most adopters had to face a degree of uncertainty or resistance in their efforts to achieve adoptive parenthood. While Ryburn's (1996) research suggests it is possible to continue direct and indirect contact with birth parents who oppose adoption, he quite reasonably argues elsewhere (1994 and 1997a) that the adversarial nature of contested proceedings makes a poor foundation on which to build co-operative contact arrangements. On the other hand, it is suggested that a willingness to negotiate with birth parents about post-adoption contact may help them to relinquish their children for adoption (Ryan 1994: 20).

Direct contact with birth mothers opposing adoption is frequently viewed as problematic because they may be less likely to give permission for adopters to assume a parenting role. However, a willingness and ability to relinquish control and responsibility is not only relevant to birth parents. Difficulties can also arise where grandparents remain hostile to adoption. For example, a single adoptive mother who adopted her daughter without parental consent described contact with grandparents as follows:

> Carol does have a need to have contact with someone from her past – someone who knew her for the first eleven years of her life – she has a need for her grandparents to try. I also felt very hurt that they obviously think I'm such a terrible person when they can see how wonderful Carol is. They would always refuse to let her call me Mum and things like that and they told me that I am not Carol's mother and that I never will be and that I was only her guardian. They don't seem to understand – I'm sure they've had adoption explained to them but they choose not to accept it.

The adopter felt it was important for contact to continue and was trying to organise a social worker to accompany Carol on contact visits. In some cases adopters were cautious about inviting grandparents to their homes, fearing that out of sympathy for birth parents they might divulge identifying information or adopters' addresses. Additionally, older children who cared for their younger siblings when they were neglected by birth parents may have difficulty in 'letting go' and trusting someone else to provide good parenting. For the past six years Karen, who was adopted by one of our sample families, had been having direct contact with her older sister Frances. The adoptive parents understood Frances's special concern for Karen but worried that she found it difficult to accept her sister's situation:

> There are problems with contact but you know Karen has said sometimes 'I'd love to live with my sister Frances'. And Frances always says to her 'I remember when you were a little baby and I used to push you in the pram' and all this, and wouldn't it be great if we were like that again. And Karen's got this idea they were all one big happy family when they were together. I think its like anything – you look back at things in your childhood and always think things were better than they were – and she doesn't remember any of the bad bits.
>
> (Adoptive father)

Issues associated with relinquishing parenting responsibilities do not necessarily constitute a sufficient reason for abandoning direct contact, but they do require attention and possible intervention for adopters to experience contact as beneficial for themselves and their adopted children.

## Managing arrangements for contact: a complicated business

As we noted in Chapter 4, arrangements for post-adoption contact experienced by the sixty-one adoptive families were so complicated and varied that they almost defy categorisation. This reflects Parker's (1999: 58) comments in his overview of ten studies funded by the Department of Health. The following discussion concentrates on direct contact, which was formally agreed between the parties prior to adoption. It demonstrates the kind of arrangements that adoptive parents had to manage even where, as in some cases, contact subsequently lapsed or was stopped. As we will see later, these formal arrangements for contact became blurred as time went on and additional birth relatives became involved.

Many adoptive families and their children were involved in contact arrangements, which included a variety of birth relatives rather than particular members of birth families only. Where *only* birth parents, grandparents from one side of the birth family or adopted siblings were involved, organising contact was relatively straightforward. While arranging contact with other siblings may appear relatively easy, this was not always the case. For example, some siblings from the same family were living in separate placements and adopters had to co-ordinate arrangements with up to four different carers to get all the children together. Other siblings were still 'looked after' by local authorities and adopters commented that social workers were too busy to arrange contact, that siblings were moved around and they did not always know where they were living and that planned meetings were often cancelled by social services. The difficulties faced by adoptive parents in maintaining contact between their children and looked-after siblings is not unique to our sample and was a cause of complaint for adopters in the study undertaken by Lowe *et al.* (1999). Arranging contact for the forty-three children in twenty-six adoptive families, where a combination of birth relatives was involved, could be problematic. When a group of birth relatives came to the same meetings this was easier in terms of time management and travelling arrangements. However, it often presented additional challenges for adopters who wanted to ensure that children and birth relatives all had an opportunity to interact and to benefit from contact. In some cases where birth relatives had not emotionally relinquished the children it was difficult for adopters to effectively supervise secret conversations and whispered remarks when several members of the birth family were present at the same time. When children were having contact with different birth relatives at separate meetings adoptive parents could find this time consuming and disruptive.

Agencies need to consider two particular issues here when they are negotiating contact arrangements. First, plans for direct and indirect contact must achieve a balance between the needs of children and birth families and allowing sufficient practical and emotional space for adoptive families to function and develop. Second, agencies should anticipate, as far as possible, birth relatives who may request or become involved in contact later and anticipate with adopters how this can be managed. These issues require agencies to confirm adoptive parents' authority to exercise discretion in relation to contact and to give them confidence in carrying out their own balancing act when the agency is no longer around to support them. One example with extremely complicated possibilities for direct and indirect contact illustrates these issues. The Brown family adopted two unrelated children. For Tom, direct post-adoption contact was agreed every six to eight weeks with his maternal grandparents. However, as time went on the grandparents began to bring Tom's two siblings to visits and they told us that they intended to ask the adoptive parents if they could also bring their other daughter's children. Tom also had two-way indirect contact with his birth mother. When Pat was subsequently adopted, direct contact was agreed with her paternal grandmother at around six times a year. Although not part of the agreement, the paternal grandmother began to bring her mother and her daughter to visits. The adopters also managed indirect two-way contact with Pat's maternal grandmother and her paternal grandfather. As Pat's birth mother's health improved she also became included in two-way indirect contact. Finally, Pat's birth mother had another baby who was placed for adoption and direct annual contact had begun with him. While Tom and Pat's adoptive parents were happy with these arrangements they said they had to do some hard thinking about what was desirable and manageable:

> We did have a lot of thinking to do about this because we didn't really want someone turning up on the doorstep once a fortnight. We had already got these visits for Tom and it was going to be paternal grandmother, paternal grandfather and maternal grandmother. So if you're going to allow six or eight visits a year all of a sudden you're going to have someone turning up every other week, which I don't think is practical in terms of a normal family life for the children – we've got our own families as well.
>
> (Adoptive mother)

Although this family had a particularly complicated package of contact arrangements, it was not uncommon for adopters to maintain direct and indirect contact with several birth relatives many of whom lived a considerable distance away.

## Direct contact: losses and gains

We noted earlier that, of the sixty-one families who had undertaken to maintain post-adoption contact, five were not in direct contact with *any* birth relatives at the time of the research. Direct contact with birth parents and other relatives was stopped for five children in two families because it was evidently destructive and damaging for the children. Indirect contact was maintained in these cases. For one family the birth mother had not contacted the adopters to arrange contact and in another, when the birth mother left a gap of several months, her son refused to see her. In the second case the child had also lost contact with a fostered and an adopted sibling, apparently because the respective adults could not sort out mutually convenient arrangements. The adoptive parents in these two families were content to allow direct contact to lapse, although indirect contact had been substituted in one family. In the final case, adoptive parents reported that the adopters of their daughter's sibling were unwilling to maintain direct contact. They were genuinely concerned about this and encouraged their daughter to phone and write to her sister although she received very little response. The adopters had also contacted the adoption agency to enlist their help. When we talked to Linda she told us how much she worried about her sister and said 'I think about her nearly every minute – what she's doing now and if she's OK.' Her hopes for the future were that she would keep in touch with her sibling and when she was able she would 'go and see her an awful lot – lots more – every weekend'. Fifteen children in a further eleven families had lost direct contact with at least one birth-family member whilst retaining contact with others. In two families, the adopters were maintaining direct contact with a birth parent in which the children were not involved. While some originally agreed contact arrangements lapsed over time, direct contact developed with other birth relatives who were not included in pre-adoption arrangements. Twenty-one (22 per cent) children in fifteen adoptive families found additional birth relatives entering their lives, including birth parents, siblings, aunts and cousins. These additional contacts largely arose as birth relatives brought other family members with them on contact visits and new siblings were born. Macaskill (2002) and Owen (1999) also note a tendency for some birth relatives, where direct contact was formally agreed at adoption, to enlarge the circle of birth-family meetings. The introduction of additional birth relatives was largely unproblematic for adopters in our sample. In only two families did this cause concern. One adoptive family felt anxious when their children's birth mother, who was excluded from direct contact, began attending local social functions and meeting with the children. In the second family, grandparents were taking the child out without the adopters and meeting up with other birth relatives for whom contact had not been agreed. The adopters did not object to this extension of contact but were upset that it was their daughter, rather than her grandparents, who told them about it.

While most pre-adoption agreements about contact remained in place, the passage of time led to some losses and some gains in direct contact between children and their birth families. However, only one adoptive family told us the adoption agency had guaranteed them a specific number of social-work hours if they needed to call on its help in relation to post-adoption contact. While some adoptive families had returned to their adoption agency for help with contact issues, they did not covey the impression that post-adoption support was a service they could call on as of right. It is clear that for the adoptive parents in our sample, adoption agencies negotiated direct-contact arrangements prior to adoption and then largely left adopters and birth-family members to get on with it. An awareness of changing circumstances over time should prompt social workers to anticipate some fluidity in contact arrangements, to prepare adoptive parents for managing this and to mediate in situations where adoptive parents or birth relatives are unable to resolve problems arising from contact arrangements.

## Adoptive parents' perceptions: advantages of direct contact

Thus far in this chapter we have considered the complexity of contact arrangements and challenges faced by adoptive parents in organising and managing meetings between children and their birth families. We now want to look at the quality and content of meetings and their impact on adopters. The following discussion will consider these issues from accounts of adoptive parents in the sixty-one sample families. One of the factors that motivates adopters to maintain direct post-adoption contact is that they think there are advantages in doing so. Adoptive parents in our sample were able to identify advantages for participants from at least one side of the adoption triangle. Adoptive parents of fifty-six children in thirty-five families (57 per cent) were able to identify advantages for themselves, their children and birth-family members. In twenty families with twenty-seven children adopters thought that, although they gained little from contact, it had advantages for their children and birth relatives. Parents in only three adoptive families with six children felt that contact had no advantages other than for birth relatives.

Three further families presented rather more complicated pictures. In one, adopters had different contact arrangements for two unrelated children. For their first child they thought contact had advantages for all concerned. However, their second child had Down's syndrome and they considered that contact was advantageous only for his birth mother. In the second family, two adopted sisters had contact with an older sibling who tended to systematically exclude one of them in favour of interacting with the other. The adopters and their teenage daughter whom we interviewed all spoke of the significant distress that this had caused. So, in this family adopters rated contact for one of their daughters as having advantages for her and her sibling but thought that, for their other daughter, any advantage was experienced only by the sibling. In the third family, contact was thought to have advantages only for the birth parents and, although it had been planned to continue post-adoption, contact stopped when an adoption order was made. The children remained in direct contact with their birth sister and the adopters saw this as having advantages for all participants. Thus, in sixty-two sets of contact arrangements (as opposed to adoptive families) there were only five cases where adopters thought that contact was exclusively to the advantage of birth relatives. In one additional family, two siblings were assessed as experiencing the advantages and disadvantages of contact quite differently.

When identifying advantages for themselves, adopters discussed the importance of access to information about their children's histories, keeping knowledge about birth relatives up to date and actively participating in conversations about birth families with their children. They did not want their children to blame them for excluding birth relatives from their lives and some felt they would be better prepared if children wanted to trace other members of their birth families when they grew up. Adopters explained:

I think with his Mum, he also knows he can talk about her with us. I mean –
he doesn't much but we'll occasionally say the name of someone and he'll
say 'oh we knew somebody called that when I was with Linda' [birth mother].
Or he'll occasionally say incidents that happened like his sister got a fork
down her throat when he was with Linda. He feels totally free to be able to
talk about it.

> (Adoptive mother: direct contact with maternal grandmother,
> birth mother and adopted siblings)

We don't want the children saying later 'you stopped us from seeing our
brother'.

> (Adoptive mother: direct contact with maternal
> grandparents and brother)

It's about knowing what makes Dave tick. We didn't find that out from the
paperwork but we can get what makes him tick from his mother – not from
information but from the feel of the whole family. Because Dave is so
complicated you have to get to know as much as you can to get inside his head.

> (Adoptive mother: direct contact with birth mother,
> siblings, maternal grandmother and aunt)

Nicholas knows who his birth mother is. If when he grows up, he wants to go
to his mother or he said 'you're not my real mother' it would hurt, but not so
much as for an adoptive mum who hadn't had open adoption.

> (Adoptive mother: direct contact with birth mother and siblings)

Adopters described the advantages for their children associated with contact.
These largely related to adopters' feelings that children need to maintain links with
their 'roots'. Children had direct access to information and when they grew up
there would be no shocks or any unexpected discovery of 'skeletons in the
cupboard'. While these aspects of contact were largely identified as advantageous
for children, it was clear that they also gave adopters some peace of mind about
their children's future well-being. Adoptive parents discussed the issues as follows:

She's always known her own family. If she has any questions they are there
for her to talk to. She doesn't have to go through us or when she is eighteen
she doesn't have to start the process of finding out about her background
because they've always been there to have contact with.

> (Adoptive mother: direct contact with birth father
> and paternal grandmother)

We don't think there is any bonding there but children are curious about their
roots and roots should not be severed.

> (Adoptive father: direct contact with birth mother
> and maternal grandmother)

We know that come their teens they're going to want to know everything and as far as we're concerned we've done nothing to stop them, we've encouraged it. And they know Anne [birth mother] as Anne, so they don't have to go knocking on people's doors to find out the past – they'll already know it won't they – they've grown up with it. We don't want the boys to have any hangups when they're older, we want them to know where they came from. Quite a few people we know who've been adopted – they've gone tracing their roots. And it can create a lot of heartache later in life. We won't have the heartache and rejection later on – because I think that's a big thing.

(Adoptive father: direct contact with birth mother,
siblings living at home and adopted siblings)

It will help the children come to terms with their adoption, it allows them to see their birth family through eyes that change as they grow up. There is no mystery, no sudden crisis of personality when they reach their teens – I really thought it was a good idea. It gives them a chance to talk about it – to see her [birth mother] as they grow older. And I think as she [adopted daughter] gets older, especially, it will help her to understand why she [birth mother] couldn't have looked after the children.

(Adoptive mother: direct contact with birth mother,
maternal grandmother and adopted siblings)

It's important she knows who her blood relatives are. It's important to a child to know her roots and it's something we're at ease with. There's a big difference between reading about your relatives and actually seeing them.

(Adoptive father: direct contact with two aunts and an uncle
and access to birth mother as soon as the child wants this)

We could go on, but we hope these examples convey something of the way in which adopters thought about the advantages of contact for their children. Adoptive parents seemed to recognise something special about separated siblings' needs for contact with each other. Their views were based, not so much on the importance of access to information or identity issues, but on the recognition of an emotional closeness that grows out of shared histories and mutually supportive relationships. Many adopters intuitively grasped messages from research about the particular quality of sibling relationships (Borland *et al.* 1998; Morrow 1998) and the sense of loss experienced by separated siblings (Whitaker *et al.* 1984; Harrison, 1999). For example:

The emphasis and importance he places on his sisters is very, very important. There is an extremely strong bond with his sisters, which we recognise. He always speaks very fondly of them . . . he hugs and kisses them . . . they pick him up. There's just a very strong bond there. They still like to see their little brother and to a certain extent the older sister mothered him and brought him up.

> (Adoptive father: direct contact with two sisters living with maternal grandmother and one with maternal aunt)

Because they all went through the same experiences and they tend to look out for each other and tend to have much more concern for each other than normal siblings would. I know that Tony was particularly concerned that Philip was safe and secure and happy.

> (Adoptive father: direct contact with a brother and sister adopted separately and a brother in foster care and indirect contact with birth parents)

The emotional side of it . . . I think it's fantastic to see them together, I'd like to see them together more. He knows he's got a sister and he knows he's got a brother. He knows she's on the end of a phone and he can contact her. He can see she's always going to be there for him and he's always going to be there for her.

> (Adoptive father: direct contact with adopted sibling and indirect contact with birth parents)

Other adoptive parents talked about the bond between siblings. An adoptive mother referred to her pleasure in seeing contact between her adopted son and his sibling and said they were 'like two peas in a pod'. Another adoptive father explained that his adopted daughter had started 'acting up' because she had not seen her brother for some time due to family illness. He reported that from the time regular contact was re-established his daughter's difficult behaviour subsided and he said 'she's happy – it's as though a little light came back in her eyes – she's seeing her brother again'. However, as we noted earlier not all adopters falling outside our sample or extended birth-family members were prepared to facilitate direct contact between separated siblings. Neither should we paint too rosy a picture of sibling contact. While adoptive parents in our sample could identify advantages for their children in maintaining sibling contact, two particular issues tended to present themselves as disadvantages for adopters. First, adopters were aware that their children worried about siblings particularly if they were not settled with a family. This sometimes led adoptive parents to shoulder the worry on behalf of their children and to emphasise the advantages of contact for birth relatives (siblings) rather than for their adopted children. For example:

> Steve has left school with no qualifications, no hopes or ambitions, no job, no hobbies, no interest in anything and without wanting to be judgemental about any of that, it isn't what we want. We don't have any ambitions for any of the children but for them to see what there is in the world, what they could or might like to do and we didn't want Steve to be undermining any of that. It was very difficult for us with Steve. We realised he had no direction, nobody sticking up for him, nobody fighting for him or encouraging him, nobody

giving him any opportunities – so do we do that or don't we do that? I can see how people get into difficult situations and start to resent the whole contact issue.

(Adoptive mother: direct contact with older sibling in care)

I think Daniel is fairly insecure and lacks confidence and this [contact] can help him have more confidence and feel more secure. I'm not sure that I see much in it for our children but there might be something in it for Daniel – and if there is, I would definitely want to continue it even if our children weren't getting much from it.

(Adoptive father: direct contact with older sibling recently adopted from care)

Second, as we will discuss later, sibling contact was sometimes experienced as difficult by adoptive parents even when they perceived it as advantageous for their children. As compared to contact with birth parents, for example, sibling contact is not necessarily an easy option. This is particularly so when siblings are looked after and adopters worry about the effects of their bad language, sexual knowledge and experience, rough and excitable behaviour and attention-seeking demands. Permanent carers in Rushton *et al.*'s study (2001: 41) expressed similar concerns. Some older siblings had been sexually abused and/or had lived with parents who were violent, mentally ill or incapacitated by alcohol and drugs. Adoptive parents feared their children might hear 'gory' details about their birth families from siblings before they considered it was appropriate to provide a more balanced account of events. Difficulties could also arise when younger adopted children had contact with older siblings with whom they had never had an opportunity to establish a meaningful relationship.

All the adopters could identify advantages of direct contact for birth relatives even when this was not matched by perceived advantages for themselves or their children. Advantages for birth siblings reflected those identified for adopted children in sibling contact with the additional advantage that looked after siblings were thought to benefit from a continuity of relationships, which were absent from their 'in care' experience. Adopters expressed a good deal of sympathy for grandparents who had lost their grandchildren through no 'fault' of their own and particularly for those grandparents who had tried to care for children in situations of parental neglect. While adoptive parents did not see contact as serving to develop a relationship between their children and adult birth relatives, they understood that parents, grandparents, aunts and uncles wanted to know the children were well and happy and did not want family links to be forgotten. One adoptive mother, whose children had direct contact with their birth father, his mother and an aunt, exemplifies similar remarks made by other adoptive parents:

And I think why it appeases Harry's [birth father] conscience, I think that's part of it, he feels better about what happened. Because finally he gave his total consent to the adoption and he really tried to get Peggy [birth mother] to do the same. He really made big efforts at the last ditch to put it right, so I think it makes him feel good. Meg [aunt] and Nana [Harry's mother], God bless them, love the girls to death, absolutely to death and for them it means they know they're OK. They can see them growing up and they're still part of their lives in some way.

It must be acknowledged that while adopters thought contact had advantages for birth relatives, this was not their main concern. Sometimes birth relatives were thought to experience an advantage at the expense of children's and/or adoptive parents' well-being and occasionally birth mothers used contact to reaffirm their status as 'real' parents and their intention to resume care of the children. The following section explores these issues in greater detail.

## Adoptive parents' perceptions: comfort and satisfaction with direct contact

Adopters' willingness and ability to identify advantages of contact are important motivational factors in the maintenance of contact arrangements. However, difficulties can develop if all participants in the adoption triangle do not experience contact as equivalently advantageous – that is, if one party's advantage is gained at another party's cost. From the perspective of adoptive parents we can explain this most effectively by reference to their comfort and satisfaction with contact arrangements. The degree of comfort reported by adopters refers to their experience of contact and relationships with birth relatives. We may distinguish here between personal comfort and parental comfort, although the two are closely related. Personal comfort may be undermined, for example, if birth relatives cannot give permission for adopters to assume a parenting role or if they act in other ways to diminish adopters' sense of confidence, security or self-worth. Parental comfort becomes eroded if adopters feel their children are unsettled or distressed by contact. In these circumstances adopters in our sample became upset for their children and wanted to do something to protect them. Feelings of satisfaction with contact refer to how far adopters assessed it as being beneficial for their children in relation to its frequency and children's needs for information, reassurance, genealogical continuity and so on.

Some adoptive parents experienced personal discomfort during contact but persevered because they were satisfied it had advantages for their children and was in their best interests. A degree of parental discomfort may be endured if adopters are satisfied that the long-term advantages of contact outweigh the short-term disadvantages for children. The maintenance of direct contact is problematic in those cases where parental discomfort is high and satisfaction is low. Adopters have to negotiate a balance in their attitudes to contact based on their experience of personal and parental comfort and satisfaction with short-term disadvantages versus long-term advantages. It is a complicated and sometimes emotionally challenging equation. It should be emphasised here that we are only concerned with aspects of comfort and satisfaction, which significantly impinged on adopters' attitudes to contact. Some adopters were irritated by birth relatives' mannerisms or attitudes and had different values or aspirations for themselves and their children. However, these were minor irritations of the sort that could be accommodated without excessive tension and they did not influence adopters' willingness to continue contact arrangements.

Table 6.1 identifies adoptive parents' reported experience of comfort and satisfaction with contact at the time of the research. Most responses from married adopters were very similar, but if one adoptive parent expressed a significant degree of discomfort or dissatisfaction in any area then both adopters were included in the appropriate category.

In the majority (67 per cent) of adoptive families, adopters were comfortable and satisfied with contact. We think that in these cases it is reasonable to conclude that contact was also experienced as beneficial by the sixty-five (68 per cent) of children involved or that it was, at least, unlikely to be damaging for them. There were no adoptive families where dissatisfaction with contact occurred unaccompanied by personal and/or parental discomfort. The single family where personal comfort and satisfaction were problematic only for the adoptive mother concerns a child with Down's syndrome, who had been placed on the understanding that there would be indirect contact with her birth parents. Subsequently, the birth parents refused to agree to adoption unless they could have direct contact. The adoptive mother felt angry, betrayed, personally distressed at contact visits and could not see any advantages in contact for her adopted child.

Adopters in four families experienced personal discomfort although they thought contact remained satisfactory in terms of meeting their children's needs. In one case discomfort arose from grandparents' interference and attempts to exercise a parental role during visits. The adoptive mother commented 'I'm a bit frightened they will try to take over so I'm not as comfortable with them'. In a second family the adopters felt an older sibling was encouraging their daughter to think life had been wonderful in her birth family and it would be better if they were all together again. The third family was only one of four families where adopters said contact was personally uncomfortable because it reminded them the child was not theirs and had been born to other parents. However, we only counted one of these families in this category because, for the others, this feeling was so fleeting that it appeared to be inconsequential. Where discomfort was presented as a significant response to the lack of a birth relationship with their child, the adoptive mother said:

> The negatives [of contact] are that we are reminded that Josh has another family and that we have to meet the person who has gone through this. It is hard to accept that he is not actually ours because we feel he is but we are still reminded that he belonged to someone else. The possibility of Josh wanting to return to her in future years is always there. We have tried to provide a loving home but that possibility is always present.
> (Direct contact with birth mother and siblings living at home)

*Table 6.1* Adopters' reported experience of personal and parental comfort and satisfaction with direct contact

| Experience **unproblematic** *on personal and parental comfort and satisfaction* | Experience **problematic** *on personal and parental comfort and satisfaction* |
|---|---|
| Parents in 41 (67%) adoptive families and 42 contact arrangements with birth families (two adoptive families had contact with two birth families for their two unrelated children where their experience for both families fell into this category) Includes 65 (68%) adopted children | Parents in 5 (8%) adoptive families (one family had contact with birth parents for their children, where their experience fell into this category, but their contact with the children's sibling was problematic only on parental comfort) Includes 9 (9%) adopted children |
| Experience **problematic** *on personal comfort*, **unproblematic** *on parental comfort and satisfaction* | Experience **problematic** *on parental comfort*, **unproblematic** *on personal comfort and satisfaction* |
| Parents in 4 (7%) adoptive families Includes 5 (5%) adopted children | Parents in 3 (5%) adoptive families and 5 contact arrangements with birth families (the two additional contact arrangements include one child whose adoptive parents' experience of contact for her unrelated adopted sibling falls into another category and three children for whom contact with a sibling falls in this category, while contact with birth parents was experienced as problematic in all three areas) Includes 6 (6%) adopted children |
| Experience **problematic** *on satisfaction*, **unproblematic** *on personal and parental comfort* | Experience **problematic** *on personal and parental comfort*, **unproblematic** *on satisfaction* |
| There were no adopters who experienced satisfaction with contact as problematic in isolation from other areas of personal and parental comfort | Parents in 4 (7%) adoptive families Includes 5 (5%) adopted children |
| Experience **problematic** *on personal comfort and satisfaction*, **unproblematic** *on parental comfort* | Experience **problematic** *on parental comfort and satisfaction*, **unproblematic** *on personal comfort* |
| Parents in one adoptive family Includes one adopted child | Parents in 3 (5%) adoptive families Includes 5 (5%) adopted children |

The adoptive father in this family echoed her comments:

> I know it's good for Josh in the long run but three times in the year he's not ours. If it does him good it's OK, it's just me feeling bad about the three hours when I feel he's not ours.

The last adopters in this group experienced personal discomfort because of particularly difficult contact arrangements. Contact did not appear to have a negative impact on their two children and they felt the potential advantages made it worth continuing. Initially contact with the maternal grandfather and birth mother had been held at a social services centre and was supervised by a social worker. Meetings subsequently moved to neutral territory and were unsupervised. The adopters reported that the birth mother disliked meeting in communal places so they agreed to meet at the grandfather's home. Visits were described as 'chaotic' with the children's birth mother wrapping up presents for them as they arrived, shouting and taking the children into the bedroom for private conversations. The adoptive mother described her feelings about this situation:

> I'm not saying she would do any harm to them but you're out of that, you've no control over what's happening, you can't hear what she's saying to them, you can't interrupt, you can't alter the situation. And you wriggle and you squirm and my husband will look at me and I'll look at him and I know he's getting himself into a state. And we have granddad sitting there and he loves seeing the children, but he finds her hard to cope with at the best of times and there's all this going on – this undercurrent, you know, and we're trying to keep an aura of normality.

Different problems were involved for adopters in the three families and five contact arrangements where parental discomfort was experienced but adopters remained satisfied that, on balance, contact continued to have advantages for their children. Parental discomfort was, however, associated with adopters' worries about their children's well-being and in four cases this arose from contact with siblings. Siblings in two of these situations were 'in care' and adopters were concerned about the impact of their immature, demanding and wild behaviour on their children. Another sibling had been sexually abused in her birth family and the adopters did not want her to tell their children about this until they felt it was appropriate to explain. Although she had been adopted by the time of the research, our sample adoptive father described this sibling as 'a bit of a wild card' who gave his children 'a hard time'. He was very sympathetic about her harrowing experiences and recognised a special sibling bond between her and his children, such that he thought contact should continue. The final arrangement caused adopters parental discomfort for rather different reasons. Their daughter was having contact with her older sister who lived with the extended family. Contact had become sporadic and unreliable because the sister tended to stay with friends and did not return the adopters' phone calls. The lack of contact was upsetting their daughter for whom the adopters felt that seeing her sister was very important. Finally, in this category, adopters had previously fostered their son and said they had witnessed his distress and resistance to contact with his birth mother. Direct contact continued post-adoption and as he got older Ted appeared to be less disturbed by his birth mother's visits. The adopters said they thought the potential advantages for Ted outweighed any short-term upset. Thus, while the adopters were satisfied with contact they also experienced parental discomfort about its impact on their son's happiness. As it happened in this case, Ted's birth mother failed to make arrangements for contact and when she finally got in touch he refused to see her. Indirect contact was substituted following the breakdown of direct contact.

In three of the four families where adopters experienced personal and parental discomfort but expressed satisfaction with contact, difficulties again arose in the context of direct contact with siblings. In two cases adopted children appeared to have complicated and ambivalent feelings about sibling contact, which we think it inappropriate to try and interpret here. One adoptive mother said of her six-year-old daughter who had contact with older siblings:

> She'd actually say and she'd tell everyone I was a naughty mummy – I took her back and I shouldn't have taken her back. She'd come back and cling more to Andy [adoptive father] because she said I'd taken her and I was horrible. She used to face me – you're a naughty mummy – you shouldn't have taken me. We tried to explain but she wouldn't have it and she sulked for a week. In future I hope that they [social workers] are right and that she will forget all those bad times and bad experiences and having the stress and that she will only remember the continuance of contact. And out of it I suppose I see a positive side for her – that she will get more of the truth and will be able to discuss, particularly with Charlie [oldest sibling], about what really happened and they could probably support each other through that.

Another adoptive mother described visits with her son to see his older adopted siblings. Sam had never lived with his siblings as they had been removed from their parents' care before his birth. The adoptive mother reported that Sam refused to get in the car when he knew they were setting off for a visit and refused to get out of the car when they arrived. During contact he sulked. She was acutely aware that Sam's siblings had their usual activities suspended for his visits only to be confronted by a child who apparently wanted nothing to do with them. This situation adversely affected the adoptive mother's personal and parental comfort with contact:

> He gets into the car saying he's not going, doesn't want to go and gets upset. He blames me for setting the contact up and then blames me for ending it – so I'm in a no-win situation.

But both adopters thought there were advantages for Sam in continuing contact:

> We felt that if Sam learned the truth as he grew up he would be able to cope with what had happened. He's got an instinctive feel that he has this family. When he talks about his brothers and sister he means his siblings, not my daughters and son. He likes the idea of having his brothers and sister and when he sees them it reinforces it because they are actually real.

Adopters in the third family were concerned about the rough and unruly behaviour of two older siblings, one fostered and one living with the extended birth family, with whom their children had contact. The adoptive mother reported their experience:

> It was when Russell was attention seeking, he wasn't happy with the environment he was in and he was very rough with Angie [adopted daughter]. And on another occasion she came away with a split lip. So we were thinking, is this what contact's always going to be like?'

The last family in this category felt their son should continue to see his birth mother and maternal grandmother to provide familial continuity, help him understand adoption and provide ongoing information about his birth relatives. Visits were arranged in a neutral place and were supervised by a worker. The adoptive mother explained the reasons for her discomfort:

> I don't like it, it makes me uncomfortable but I don't feel threatened by it, nor do I feel my position as Ben's parent is threatened by it. It's just who might be there and what horrible things might happen and what she [Freda, the birth mother] might say to Ben to upset him. Freda isn't a problem but those amongst her are. She's not very bright and she's very volatile and emotional and if she had a step-dad with her or a natural dad they could create an awful problem and it wouldn't be an exaggeration to say they would pick him up and go. I always go in with Ben to try to ease him in. At first as I walked through the door his grandmother used to grab him off me and close the door behind her. Ben got quite upset so now I always try to get there first so we can be there ready and she can come in and do her hellos and her crying and everything with him. Then we make small talk for a little while and then I go and sit in the room across the corridor.

Although the adopters could see long-term advantages for Ben, his birth mother's inability to relinquish him to his new family led her to say things that confused him. His adoptive mother reported 'last time he was very upset by it all and even three or four weeks after he was asking ''I am your boy aren't I?'''

The adopters we have discussed thus far decided to maintain direct contact because they thought any discomfort or short-term problems were outweighed by long-term advantages for their children. However, in two categories where one or both forms of adult discomfort were *accompanied by dissatisfaction with contact*, the maintenance of contact was extremely difficult and in some families it had stopped. In the five families where adopters experienced problems in all three areas and the three families where they expressed parental discomfort and dissatisfaction with contact, children were having contact with birth mothers in four cases and with birth fathers in two. All birth mothers had contested their children's adoption while the birth fathers had agreed. Although in three of these six families it was intended that direct contact should continue post-adoption, the courts found that this would not be in the children's best interests and it was stopped for two birth mothers and one father. Children in two of these families made it clear that they were distressed by contact and did not want it to continue. The two birth mothers involved here were adamantly opposed to adoption. Adopters reported that they tried to undermine the placements by telling their children they should continue to use their birth names, the adopters were not their real parents and that they were fighting to get them home. A further birth mother had failed to contact the adopters to make arrangements for seeing her son. In this case the adoptive mother, who had begun as a foster carer, was very relieved about the birth mother's disappearance from the scene as she felt contact had been extremely distressing for her son and for herself. In two further families involving birth parents, contact was continuing. Both of these families had begun by fostering their children, post-adoption contact was frequent and somehow the adopters had struggled on until their children were old enough to make their own arrangements for visits. The adopters here seemed powerless to act on their own assessment of contact's relative advantages and disadvantages for their children. However, we do know from talking to one of these children, who was 12 years old, that he had to manage many problematic aspects of contact arrangements on behalf of the adults involved. His situation is discussed in greater detail in Chapter 9. The other two families in this category, where contact was ongoing, were meeting with maternal grandparents and a sibling respectively and we have referred to their difficulties earlier in this chapter. Grandparents disapproved of the adoptive mother, refused to have her at contact visits, told her she was not her daughter's real parent and were opposed to their granddaughter's adoption. Problems arose for the family having sibling contact because one of their daughters was distressed by what she experienced as rejection and exclusion during visits when the adult sibling favoured her sister. Of these eight problematic contact situations, five occurred in families approved for adoption and three in families who had initially fostered their children.

An analysis of particular birth relatives with whom children were having contact suggests that adoptive parents experienced birth- parent contact as most problematic. If we consider the numbers of birth relatives in each group, adopters expressed variations of parental and personal discomfort and dissatisfaction in response to 29 per cent of contacts with birth parents, 24 per cent with siblings and 22 per cent with grandparents. This looks rather different if we only take into account adoptive parents' reports of dissatisfaction with contact because they thought the disadvantages outweighed any advantages for their children. In this case adopters felt dissatisfied with 29 per cent of birth-parent contacts, 13 per cent of grandparent contacts and only 3 per cent of sibling contacts. This indicates again that satisfaction with contact can be experienced alongside personal and parental discomfort and, while sibling contact can cause discomfort, adopters felt in the vast majority of cases that it was advantageous for their children and should be maintained.

We noted earlier in this chapter that respondents who originally fostered their children were not necessarily more comfortable with post-adoption contact. Of all adoptive parents expressing various combinations of discomfort and dissatisfaction with contact, 33 per cent had initially been approved as prospective adopters and

37 per cent had acted as foster carers for their children. Of those who felt dis-satisfied with contact, 16 per cent had previously been foster carers and 14 per cent had started out as prospective adopters. Where contact was with birth parents, there was no difference between these two groups in their experience of parental consent to adoption. Our analysis of interviews with adoptive parents suggests that motivational factors are significant here. Foster carers, just as much as prospec-tive adopters, wanted children to be their own and by the time of adoption had developed strong parental feelings towards them. It is a mistake to assume that because foster carers are expected to facilitate pre-adoption contact they will experience fewer difficulties when contact is continued after adoption. Post-adoption, foster carers turn into parents and, as we discuss below, parenthood introduces a whole new meaning into family relationships.

## Ownership, control and direct contact

As we have explained, advocates for post-adoption contact tend to argue that the way in which law and society approach parenthood and adoption can act to frustrate continuing contact. Adoptive parents are encouraged to think about their children as if they had been born to them and the law supports this perspective through a 'legal fiction' and a refusal to interfere with adopters' exercise of parental respon-sibility. This understanding conspires to negate the post-adoption significance of birth families and empowers adopters to control the extent to which they may play any role in children's futures. Our interviews with adopters confirm this view of adoptive parenthood. However, for our sample the characteristics of adoptive parenthood acted to facilitate rather than to impede direct contact in the vast majority of cases. Nearly all adopters wanted the legal security and permanence afforded by adoption. Even when children had initially been fostered, only seven of the nineteen former foster families said they would have been happy to continue fostering although, under these circumstances, they would have wanted a guarantee of permanence.

However, it was clear from our interviews that adoption achieves far more than legal security – it constructs parenthood. It was the experience and meaning of parenthood – legally, socially and emotionally – that was of enormous significance to the adopters in our sample. For many adoptive parents the phenomenology of parenthood is intrinsically characterised by a sense of ownership and control – those very features of adoption that some advocates of contact wish to dismantle. In answer to an open-ended question about what features of adoption were important to them, at least one adoptive parent in forty-nine (83 per cent) families spontaneously identified factors associated with 'ownership' of their children. They explained this as follows:

> Because the children would be legally mine, legally mine, just as if they had been born to me. I'm just used to it now – they're just my kids. I don't even think they're adopted – they are just my kids.
>     (Adoptive mother: direct contact with maternal grandparents and brother)

Just because the children are ours. I don't even think about it now – I just know they are our kids and that's it – we are a family.

(Adoptive father: direct contact with maternal grandmother, birth mother and adopted siblings)

So that you feel he's absolutely yours – I wanted to feel that he was really ours. We are his parents. Adoption really made him ours.

(Adoptive mother: direct contact with birth mother and 'looked-after' siblings)

Two particular themes emerged from adopters' discussion of ownership. First, as they explained it, ownership is not just about 'possessing' children but incorporates a strong sense of belonging that is expressed through family relationships:

But you just look at her and fall in love. She's that sort of child. We just wanted her – she was part of us. She's ours now and we've got her. Once she's adopted she's ours. It's just like a normal family then isn't it?

(Adoptive father: direct contact with birth mother and adopted siblings)

The problem of belonging – of us all belonging as a family. Ann did get confused before the actual court hearing. She used to have to be tucked up tightly in bed every night. On the night we came back from the adoption she said 'I don't need being tucked up now – I belong'. I don't think if we had been long-term fostering we would have had the safety and deep belonging – I don't think you ever get that without adoption.

(Adoptive mother: direct contact with maternal grandmother and adult sister)

Second, adopters explained how the relationship between ownership and parenthood incorporates a responsibility to protect and care for their children. This brings with it a personally experienced and often unexpected pain that anyone could have harmed them:

It helps deep down inside yourself to know the child is yours and to treat him as yours. I can relax and give him every bit of love, care and help I want to, knowing he won't be taken away. It's security for me and for him also. You need that if you're willing to give the child your unconditional love. You have to have the security of knowing he's yours.

(Adoptive mother: direct contact with birth mother, her new baby and 'looked-after' siblings)

When I actually came to the contact I was surprised how hard it actually was. I wasn't expecting it to be that hard but when we did the contact we had had the children three months and, instead of it being theoretical, they were my children. And it really came home to me that these were the people who had been cruel to my children.

> (Adoptive mother: direct contact with maternal grandmother,
> birth mother and adopted siblings)

It's very difficult because I can answer this from my head and I can answer it from my heart. In my head I'm sympathetic for all the people concerned – everyone. But I cannot forgive, in my heart I can't forgive them for what they allowed to happen. Because, I mean even after Carol, we actually went through to court and she was legally mine, you know through the court, then my attitude changed again really in that she was really, really mine and how could anyone do this to my daughter and how could anyone betray her.

> (Adoptive mother: direct contact with maternal grandparents
> and indirect contact with birth mother)

I got to the stage where I was physically sick at some of the things they [the children] were telling us because by that stage they were our children. And I was very angry with social services because they knew about the abuse and they kept the family together for another two years – so the children had another two years of abuse after the first awareness of things. I find that hard to accept – my lack of power.

> (Adoptive mother: direct contact with birth parents was terminated
> at adoption but continued with the children's birth sister)

At least one parent in thirty-six (61 per cent) families specifically emphasised control over decision-making as an important characteristic that differentiates adoption from other arrangements. The value that adopters placed on control is clearly related to their sense of ownership. They described this in the following ways:

> Well, having short-term children really made us realise that none of them can be yours – you know, you're nobody really. None of the decisions about anything at all – where they go to school, what they do – anything – it's not your decision. Not being able to fight for what they need the way you can for your own child and yet it's even more important.

> (Adoptive mother: direct contact with sister for one child and
> birth mother and brother for second unrelated child)

From that time on they're your family. If I say one word that summed up the whole situation with contact as well – we are in control and that is so vital.

> (Adoptive mother: direct contact with maternal grandfather
> and birth mother)

If you are not going to be 100 per cent a parent you are just minding somebody for someone else and looking over your shoulder the whole time. A carer is judged on anything they do – are the children too fat, too thin, can I cut their hair – their nails. If that's your child it's up to you. But it's hard being a parent who is not 100 per cent a parent.

> (Adoptive mother: direct contact with maternal grandmother,
> birth mother and two adult sisters)

Adoption is remarkably powerful, not only in its legal effects, but in the way it operates to construct new phenomenological identities and relationships. For our adopters, the experience of ownership and control expresses a complex 'package' of attributes, which characterise parenthood and which can only be achieved through adoption. The perceived relationship between parenthood and 'family belonging' was also apparent with at least one adopter in twenty-seven (46 per cent) families emphasising the creation of a family as an important consequence of adoption. What is particularly noteworthy in the context of this discussion is the way in which ownership and control served to facilitate the maintenance of direct contact. Many adoptive parents explained the relationship between these characteristics of adoptive parenthood and contact:

I think we can be magnanimous because we are his parents, because we are secure in our position, we are his parents.

> (Adoptive mother: direct contact with birth mother,
> adopted sibling and 'looked-after' sibling)

It gives firm boundaries of knowing who, ultimately, has control. We might have managed without it but may not have felt so certain or been prepared to be so open and liberal if we hadn't known that we had the decision making power and the authority to alter arrangements. We've probably shown a lot more trust because we know we have the power to alter things.

> (Adoptive father: direct contact with maternal grandmother,
> birth mother and adopted siblings)

Because I'm the parent – the responsible party. I'm the father now and as far as I'm concerned we have the legal power now.

> (Adoptive father: direct contact with birth mother and
> siblings living with her)

I think it's because when we got the adoption order we got control over the situation. We can go back and say we think we've got a problem – let's do something about it. If we hadn't got the adoption order I just don't think we'd be able to do that. They are my children and I make the decisions – they're mine and always will be.

> (Adoptive mother: direct contact with older
> adopted sibling)

It gives you that confidence, the fact that they are legally yours. It's like having an insurance policy – you haven't actually got to call on it – but it's nice to have it in the background. It makes you much more relaxed.

(Adoptive father: direct contact with maternal grandparents)

For us it means the kids are ours. It actually makes you feel in a stronger position. You have got that thing at the end of the day – you can turn round and just say 'no – forget it' because of the adoption order. You've got the power, you've got the reins. We can act in the best interests of our children.

(Adoptive father: direct contact with older sibling living with
birth mother and indirect contact with birth mother)

I certainly feel a lot more comfortable at contact now – we are in command.

(Adoptive mother: direct contact with maternal grandparents,
'looked-after' siblings and indirect contact with birth mother)

Other studies have also found that an ability to control contact arrangements is important to adoptive parents (Barth and Berry 1988; Fratter 1996; Grotevant and McRoy 1998). In this context it is unsurprising to find that adopters in fifty-three (87 per cent) of our sample families did not want contact to be regulated or imposed by a court order. Six of the eight adopters who expressed a preference for legal regulation did so because they thought it would ensure the continuation of contact and would provide clear boundaries for those involved. Two adopters wanted an order to enforce contact, one with his son's adopted sibling with whom contact had been lost and the other with a sibling 'in care' where the local authority repeatedly cancelled meetings. Confusion about contact obligations is also of some interest in this connection. We can confirm that courts made contact orders alongside adoption orders under section 8 of the Children Act 1989 for four children placed in four adoptive families. However, adopters in nine families quite erroneously thought contact orders had been made and adopters in two families thought their arrangements were informal when information from social workers indicated their children's adoptions were accompanied by orders for contact. Adopters' confusion over the legal status of contact arrangements has been identified elsewhere (Macaskill 2002). This may be exacerbated by different agency policies about the degree of formality that should be built into contact agreements and the extent to which they should be incorporated in written agreements (Lowe *et al.* 1999).

We also explained to adopters in our sample that the government intended to introduce a special form of guardianship through the Adoption and Children Bill (now the Adoption and Children Act 2002). This would provide permanence, give guardians 'parental responsibility' and the authority to make decisions in respect of children but would not, as adoption does, deprive birth parents of parental responsibility. In answer to our question about whether they would consider caring for a child under these arrangements, forty-six (78 per cent) adoptive mothers and thirty-two (65 per cent) adoptive fathers said they would not. Ten (17 per cent) adoptive mothers and twelve (25 per cent) adoptive fathers said it would depend on factors like the birth parents' attitude to someone else looking after their child, the reasons for care away from birth families and the degree of control they would have in making decisions. Only one adoptive mother and two adoptive fathers were able to give an unequivocal 'yes' to this question. The remainder of adoptive parents did not provide sufficiently clear answers for categorisation. Now, it is unsurprising that people who are motivated to adopt should reject an arrangement that does not meet their requirements for establishing parenthood. However, their reasons for taking this view consistently reflect their perception that Special Guardianship would not afford them that degree of ownership and control which is achieved through adoption. They said for example:

> The child needs to know what the future holds and if they are not adopted it would be a case of 'I'm caring for you but your name is still somebody else's name'. It's like sitting on the edge of your chair for ten, twenty, thirty years and it's not being part of a family – it's being a visitor. I wouldn't go for that. There's bound to be conflict for the simple fact that one family – for whatever reason – has had to let go of the child and another family has taken on that child. Nobody would feel safe in that situation – it would be too complicated.
>
> (Adoptive mother: direct contact with maternal grandmother, birth mother and siblings)

> I think it would cause a lot of upset. One of the difficulties for me would be the feeling that the child isn't really ours.
>
> (Adoptive father: direct contact with birth mother and adopted siblings)

> I don't know, I just can't see it working. It would make me feel insecure – it's bound to. Although these children are with you permanently, you still haven't got the last decision to make, be it something like wanting to emigrate to Australia or . . . you're not totally in control and that's one thing about adoption – you've got control and security.
>
> (Adoptive mother: direct contact with older adopted sister)

> It is just the fear of not being in control.
>
> (Adoptive father: direct contact with paternal grandmother, aunt, great grandmother and sibling for one child, and maternal grandparents and siblings for the second child. Indirect contact with birth mothers for both children)

The significant point here is not so much adopters' understanding (or mis-understanding) of Special Guardianship, but the way in which their response to this proposal emphasises and re-affirms two vitally important issues. First, while Special Guardianship conveys parental responsibility it does not construct parent-hood. Second, and closely related to the first point, adopters could not believe that Special Guardianship would bestow a sufficient degree of ownership and control to enable effective parenting, security and stability for the child while birth parents retained parental responsibility.

## Conclusion

It is evident that many adoptive parents in our sample were managing complicated contact arrangements. They were prepared to maintain contact, sometimes under difficult circumstances, for as long as they thought it had some long-term advantage for their children. We could identify only two cases where adopters' attitudes may have negatively affected birth mothers' willingness and ability to maintain agreed contact *after* adoption. These families were discussed earlier where one birth mother delayed contact and her son finally refused to see her and the other did not initiate contact with the adopters. In the latter case the adopters had previously fostered their son and his adoptive mother said:

> From our point of view I'm glad he doesn't see his mother now. I couldn't cope with him coming back as distressed as he was after the last contact. If he did start seeing her again I'd be worried all the time – I wouldn't want him to move off my knee or let her touch him. I know it sounds selfish and horrible but I don't want to share him with anyone. I'm his mum. I looked after him and got him up in the night when it was necessary. It was me who cuddled him, took him to school, did the things mums do until you can do things capably on your own. She [birth mother] never did that, she totally neglected him and never was a real mum to him.

However, adopters in sixteen (26 per cent) families were honest enough to say they sometimes wished they did not have direct contact with birth families. It is important to understand that adopters here were describing a wish and not an intention to stop contact. They remained primarily motivated by perceived advantages and by their initial agreement to maintain contact arrangements. One adoptive mother captures the feelings expressed by others:

> We put up with it to be honest for the children. If we had a choice or if the children didn't benefit from it we would stop it to-morrow but we've still got to be open minded because of the children. Although there wasn't a court order, we said we would maintain the situation as long as it was beneficial for the children.
>
> (Direct contact with maternal grandparents and 'looked-after'
> siblings and indirect contact with birth mother)

The adoptive parents in our sample are not saints! They complained about the practical and emotional burdens imposed by contact arrangements. For example, they frequently had to take time off work and to assume responsibility for organising visits and travelling. When children were younger they had to entertain birth relatives until the children were old enough to develop relationships for themselves.

Contact visits were initially often arranged at children's birthdays and at Christmas and adopters felt this intruded on special family occasions. Birth relatives sometimes arrived at visits with mountains of gifts, some of which adopters felt were inappropriate. Contact introduced a range of issues that adoptive parents had to consider. They were concerned, for example, about their children missing a grandparent's funeral where other birth relatives would be present and about whether they should invite birth relatives to important family occasions. One adoptive mother explained her feelings in this way:

> It's another set of people to think about and to take their needs into account and it's not a set that would come naturally. It's easy for us to think we are having a birthday party and we'll invite our parents because it's the natural thing to do. But to think there is another set of people who are not part of our natural family and we have no reason to know them apart from the children . . . it's something extra to think about – how to do it in the best way to meet everyone's needs. I believe it is the right thing to do and in the long term it will benefit the children.
>
> (Direct contact with maternal grandparents and 'looked-after' sibling)

Sometimes adopters expressed resentment that they did all the hard work involved in parenting while birth relatives reaped the rewards of contact arrangements. One adoptive mother, who showed every indication of being committed to contact, said:

> It would have been perfection except that you've just got this little element and it will always be with us and we've just got to cope with it. And in some ways you think well we're doing all the everyday, nitty-gritty, routine things, running around after the children, going to the park, things at school, making sure they're growing up well, that they're doing their homework, they're developing properly. We're doing the disciplining and nurturing and for one day every three or four months all that's thrown out of the door and they get this wonderful woman who comes along like Mother Christmas and gives them lots of presents and lots of fuss.
>
> (Direct contact with birth mother and maternal grandfather)

Adoptive parents in our sample are not unique in raising these issues and similar concerns have been identified in other studies (Lowe *et al.* 1999; Macaskill 2002; Neil 2002b). However, even when adopters felt that contact imposed additional burdens we found, as did Fratter (1996), that the majority of adoptive parents were open and generous in their attitudes to birth relatives and the importance of maintaining contact for their children.

At various points in this chapter we have commented on the role of social workers in arranging and supporting direct post-adoption contact. It is evident from adoptive parents' experiences that agencies and social workers appeared to be largely concerned with negotiating contact arrangements and not with their longer-term consequences. Post-adoption, adoptive parents and birth relatives were left to manage contact as best they could. While we do not know whether and how social workers prepared birth relatives for ongoing contact, concerns expressed by adoptive parents suggest that some birth relatives had not accepted the children's adoptive situations and did not understand the purpose of contact and their role in the children's lives. We also suspect a lack of clarity about the relationship between adoption and the purpose of continuing contact. For example, if contact is about maintaining birth-family links and helping children to incorporate their history, present and future into their developing sense of identity, we can see no good reason for locating contact visits at Christmas and birthdays when this can create tensions for adoptive families. Social workers, children's guardians and the courts need to recognise that establishing contact arrangements is only the beginning of a long and evolving process where all participants require adequate preparation and support.

Some of these problems have been noted by the Social Services Inspectorate, which found post-adoption support to be 'underdeveloped and poorly advertised' (Department of Health 2000: 64). The Inspectorate identified a widespread failure to review contact arrangements and expressed concern about social workers promoting contact primarily for the benefit of birth parents. There are clear messages from our own research, other studies and the Department of Health about the necessity for improving policy and practice in relation to post-adoption contact. Sustainable contact arrangements also require government's plans for better post-adoption support (Department of Health 2002c) to incorporate services that are flexible, sensitive and readily available. Neil (2002b: 22) similarly concludes from her research:

> What led to successful, sustained contact, were arrangements that reflected the aims of contact and supported people who needed support without assuming complications where there were not any.

## Summary

- Of the adoptive parents in our sixty-one families, forty-two (69 per cent) had been approved as prospective adopters and nineteen had initially acted as foster carers for the children they subsequently adopted. Thirty (71 per cent) of the prospective adopters wanted to adopt because of infertility problems. We identified only a very small number of adoptive parents who chose adoption for purely altruistic reasons.
- Of the sixty-one adoptive families who agreed to maintain direct post-adoption contact, five were not in contact with any of their children's birth relatives at the time of the research. Fifteen children in a further eleven families had lost contact with at least one birth relative while maintaining contact with others. However, twenty-one children in fifteen families had developed new contacts as time went on.
- Where post-adoption contact continued for at least one birth relative, adoptive

parents of fifty-six children in thirty-five (57 per cent) families identified advantages of direct contact for all three sides of the adoption triangle – themselves, their children and birth relatives. In twenty families with twenty-seven children, adopters thought contact had advantages for their children and birth relatives, although it had none for them. Adopters in three families with six children felt only the birth relatives benefited from contact.

- We analysed adopters' perceptions of direct contact in relation to their feelings of personal comfort, parental comfort and satisfaction about its advantages for their children. Adoptive parents in only five families (involving 9 per cent of children) identified problems in all three areas of comfort and satisfaction. Adopters in a further three families experienced parental comfort and satisfaction as problematic and another adoptive mother expressed personal discomfort and dissatisfaction in relation to contact. We could identify only two families where adopters' attitudes may have dissuaded birth mothers from maintaining agreed contact after adoption. Adopters in one of these families expressed personal and parental discomfort with contact and in the other they found contact problematic in all three areas of comfort and satisfaction.

- Adoptive parents' perceptions of the relationship between adoption, parenthood, ownership and control served to facilitate, rather than to impede, the maintenance of direct contact. The majority of adopters opposed the imposition of a contact order and preferred to retain control over contact arrangements.

- It appears that adoption agencies were largely concerned with negotiating and establishing contact without anticipating the fluidity and complexity of ongoing arrangements. Adoptive families and birth relatives were left to get on with managing contact as best they could once an adoption order was made.

# 7 Birth relatives and direct contact

## Introduction: birth relatives, adoption and contact

We now know quite a lot about the reactions of birth mothers who request adoption for their children. While it is not the case for all relinquishing birth mothers, research indicates that many suffer an intense and prolonged sense of loss and grief (Winkler and Van Keppel 1984; Bouchier *et al.* 1991; Howe *et al.* 1992; Hughes and Logan 1993; Wells 1993). As adoption has developed into a service for looked-after children who cannot return to live with their birth parents, researchers and agencies have become more concerned with the needs of birth mothers who oppose adoption for their children. These mothers not only lose their children against their wishes, but they are additionally burdened with a social and judicial assessment that they are unfit to be parents. Mason and Selman (1998: 275) discuss the importance of providing a service for non-relinquishing birth parents who 'felt that no one in Social Services had any interest in them once their children had been removed so that most felt angry, guilty and useless'. Research suggests that birth mothers who refuse their agreement to adoption or who contest adoption applications frequently experience similar feelings to those reported by relinquishing birth mothers (Hughes and Logan 1993; Mason and Selman 1997 and 1998; Charlton *et al.* 1998; Crank 2002). Robinson (2000 and 2002) suggests that birth mothers suffer from disenfranchised grief in the sense that the loss of a child through adoption does not attract the same acknowledgement, sympathy and support as other experiences of loss. As we explain in Chapter 8, researchers have also been interested in the nature of sibling relationships and the incidence and consequences of separation for siblings who become looked after by local authorities or placed for adoption (Mullender 1999).

Although it has taken some time for researchers and practitioners to understand the relationship between adoption, loss and grief for birth mothers and siblings, we are much further behind in respect of birth fathers' responses to adoption. Birth fathers' feelings about adoption and the loss of their children have received scant attention although Deykin *et al.* (1988) in the USA and Cicchini (1993) in Australia have conducted research in this area. Clapton (2001 and 2003) reports from his research in the UK that many birth fathers experience feelings of loss, grief, anger and guilt when their children are adopted in much the same way as birth mothers. Birth grandparents come even further down the scale of attention, even though it may be argued that adoption leaves them with a double dose of loss. Grandparents not only lose frequently close and affectionate relationships with their grand-children, but also their expectations and hopes for their children as happy and competent parents who can project family continuity into the future. The Children Act 1989 gives no special recognition to grandparents and their status does not afford them an automatic right to apply for any section 8 orders or for contact with a looked-after child under section 34 of the Act. Additionally, in *Z County Council v R* [2001] 1 FLR 365, it was held that local authorities do not have a legal duty to consult members of a child's extended family when they are arranging adoptions. Grandparents may be an important resource, which enables local authorities to consider placing looked-after children with a relative, as they are required to do under section 23(6)(b) of the Children Act (Pitcher 2002). At the same time, however, grandparents are relatively disadvantaged if they want to maintain contact with their grandchildren while they are looked after, following their child's divorce or separation and after adoption. Given this situation, The Grandparents' Federation was established to campaign for arrangements that support continuing relationships between grandparents and their grandchildren and to provide help and advice for grandparents who are deprived of contact (*Family Law*, 32, 2002: 585). We hope our study will cast a little more light on birth relatives' responses to adoption and their experience of direct post-adoption contact.

From our total sample of adoptive families, we were able to interview those birth relatives who had direct-contact arrangements with thirty-two children in twenty-one families. These include six mothers, two fathers, eighteen grandparents, five aunts and an uncle, and eleven siblings who were not adopted by families in our sample and who were either looked after or living independently. In this chapter we provide an overview of these birth relatives' attitudes to adoption and their experience of direct post-adoption contact. Readers will meet some of them again in subsequent chapters when we consider children's perspectives and compare per-ceptions between adopters, children and birth relatives in triangular relationships.

## Birth relatives' attitudes to adoption and satisfaction with adoption outcome

It might be anticipated that, depending on their relationship with adopted children, birth relatives will have different attitudes towards adoption and perceptions of contact. Of the six birth mothers in this sub-sample, four were initially opposed to adoption for their children who were subject to care orders because of abuse or neglect. Two refused their agreement to the local authority's application for a freeing order and one contested an adoption application. One birth mother finally gave her agreement to adoption after months of opposition while remaining very distressed about losing her children. These mothers expressed feelings of anger and distress about their children's adoption. They said:

> Looking back I let social services walk all over me. One of my children was
> a baby suffering with colic and he cried and cried. And the social worker said

she would take him away for the weekend so I could have a break. When he was brought back he was no better and she made a report out stating that she had to take him off me and that went against me. That was the kind of crap that I've been having all these years. I was really angry at first because I wasn't heard. Whatever social services said went – I didn't get a say. The judge wasn't on my side at all – I was a bad woman who was a neglectful parent.

(Birth mother who contested adoption order)

They'd be pushing all this on me and I'd be thinking 'oh my, it's too much for me, I can't cope'. But I didn't have the bottle to say because I didn't want them to think I was not caring for them properly. I wanted more help from them instead of them taking them away – just a bit more leeway. I mean when they were with foster parents I was seeing them every day, so I wasn't getting that break. I wanted to be with them, I wanted them at home but I needed the break at the same time.

(Birth mother who finally agreed to adoption order)

My life had changed totally when they were adopted, I'd met my husband, we'd got married, we'd moved, I was a changed person. I would have been able to cope. Yes, I know I would have done. My husband has supported me all the way through – he's there for me. The other one was never there.

(Birth mother who refused her agreement to a freeing order)

The social workers decided about adoption. I got upset and told them I wanted them at home but it didn't happen.

(Birth mother who refused her agreement to a freeing order)

When we talked to them, all four birth mothers said they had come to accept their children's adoption and they no longer felt angry or resentful about social services' intervention. It was clear that seeing their children happy and well settled with adoptive families had helped them to adjust their feelings about adoption. Maintaining direct contact was crucially instrumental in birth mothers' ability to check on the well-being of their children and to feel they had not lost their parental connection. However, our conversations with these birth mothers suggested that in three cases their acceptance of adoption was ambivalent and they had not been able or willing to relinquish their emotional role as the children's birth parents. Despite this, two birth mothers and their children's adopters had managed to develop a sufficiently good working relationship to maintain direct contact. The children in these three families expressed sadness and unhappiness associated with separation from their birth mothers and/or contact. We explore these issues in greater depth in Chapters 8 and 9. The remaining birth mother unequivocally accepted that adoption was best for her children despite her earlier refusal to consent to a freeing order. She nevertheless still had a keen sense of loss three years after her children were placed for adoption:

I sometimes get upset, especially Christmas day when there is no mess through them opening their presents. I sometimes sob my heart out. I'm all right when I'm seeing them, but on the way home I break down and start crying.

Two birth mothers requested adoption for their children who had Down's syndrome. At the time of adoption one mother was sure that she was making the right decision. The other was much more ambivalent but felt she had no realistic alternative because of her family circumstances. Both mothers made strikingly similar remarks about their feelings of guilt and their reactions to seeing their children being parented by someone else:

I felt terrible, I felt guilty giving him away. It is the right decision, I don't regret it now, but I did in the beginning. I regretted what I did but I don't now. I just sort of think that I couldn't cope looking after him. I mean I still think about him, I still miss him, but that's his family now. In the beginning when I went to see him I'd want to fetch him home, but I don't feel like that now. At first it felt awful, it was really horrible. I didn't want to go away from him but it's not so bad now.

The birth mother who had felt sure about her decision was still distressed by the adoption:

I knew what my capabilities were and I knew how I was feeling when I had him adopted. It broke my heart and it still does. The first few times I saw him after his adoptive mum took him away it was terrible and I got to the stage where I said 'I don't know if I can cope with this'. I was so upset the first few times it just broke me up. I wrote to April [adoptive mother] telling her I loved seeing him but for days after I felt guilty. I wanted to see him but I didn't want the hurt. For all of two years after him being placed I had to see him but I didn't want to feel the guilt and I didn't want to get upset, but I'm fine now.

Continuing contact and the passage of time had clearly helped these mothers come to believe that adoption was best for their children. Both mothers had good relationships with the adoptive parents and, by the time of the study, they were able to relax and enjoy their contact visits without the debilitating effects of grief and guilt.

The two birth fathers having direct contact were unmarried. However, both supported the adoption plan and, while one father was instrumental in persuading the birth mother to agree to adoption after months of resistance, the other birth mother contested the order. Direct contact had served to confirm the birth fathers' views that adoption was best for their children as they saw them growing up in happy and settled environments. One father, like the relinquishing birth mothers above, described how visiting and leaving his son became easier over time:

We talk about railways and everything and it's brilliant. The thing is I don't like to stay too long because I've got myself into the situation where I don't want to upset myself, so that hour is just enough for me. It was very hard to go but it's got easier now. At first it was very hard to walk away, saying 'goodbye' and knowing I wasn't going to see him for months, but I've got over that and we've been going on for four years now.

The eighteen birth grandparents who agreed to talk to us comprised three maternal grandmothers, two paternal grandmothers, one maternal grandfather, four sets of maternal grandparents and two sets of paternal grandparents. Many of these grandparents had accommodated their grandchildren on and off in circumstances where the children were being abused and/or neglected at home. They had fed them, bought them clothes, comforted them, worried about them and tried to co-operate with social services in securing them better futures. Seven grandparents were initially opposed to adoption but only one maternal grandmother wanted her grandchildren to be returned to the care of their birth mother. One set of maternal grandparents wanted their grandchild to be placed with the extended family and a further four grandparents argued that their grandchildren should have been placed with long-term foster carers rather than adopters. However, by the time of our study all eighteen grandparents felt, in retrospect, that adoption had been the best plan and they expressed their satisfaction with the outcome. As with birth parents, direct contact enabled grandparents to maintain a sense of connection with the children and provided reassurance about their well-being. Grandparents said, for example:

Sean is happy there, the family seem to love him. He's safe and secure and he's really loved there. It helps me seeing him. I like to see him and know he's doing all right. I feel better seeing him than just speaking to him on the phone.
(Maternal grandmother initially opposed to adoption)

Seeing the children now I don't think I would want anything else. The children know the situation, my daughter knows the situation. She still sees them and so do I and we're happy with that. The children are happy and settled and we get on with their adoptive parents. I would rather have them where they are now than in a foster home not knowing whether they are staying there, going home or maybe moved to another foster home.
(Maternal grandmother initially opposed to adoption)

I agreed to them being adopted because they would be safer. We couldn't take them, we were too old to take all of the children, so when the idea of adoption came up I agreed and so did my husband – not as emphatically as me, but I said they deserved proper parents and their life would be stable. We're OK now. I know they are safe and happy and that satisfies me as long as they don't forget their nana and granddad.
(Maternal grandmother who agreed with adoption)

Well, we'd have liked to see them go to long-term foster care, but they said no they couldn't do that, it cost too much or something. Well, now I think it's very good. The children have progressed so much, they're happy and they don't swear like they used to, the language those children used to use was diabolical. They've got good parents, they've found a good couple. We still love them and it's hard for all of us, but I'm happy because they're happy.

(Paternal grandmother initially opposed to adoption)

Given that post-adoption contact had been arranged for them, it is not surprising to find that the four aunts and an uncle in this sub-sample had been closely involved in earlier adoption planning. Their accounts indicate that they had struggled with the possibility of caring for children within their extended families and had involved themselves in discussions with social services about planning and appropriate prospective adopters. A maternal aunt of three children, whose birth mother was dead, felt that she and the children's maternal grandfather had been involved in the choice of adoptive parents:

I don't know if they [social services] were letting us pretend we were involved but we actually had a meeting with the adopters. They came over here one evening and we were all here, and it must have been a terrible strain for them to come over here and be like quizzed. But we knew immediately when they came in that they were lovely people and it wasn't a problem, but we weren't going to pass the boys over to someone if we weren't sure about them. We felt we could actually have some kind of veto. Whether we could or not I don't know.

The aunts and uncle had all felt adoption was best for the children and, when we talked to them, they confirmed their satisfaction with the children's happiness and well-being. All had good relationships with adoptive parents and direct contact was reported as beneficial for all concerned.

Seven of the eleven birth siblings having direct contact, who had not been adopted by families in our sample, were old enough to remember the circumstances surrounding social services intervention and to express their views about adoption. Six siblings felt that adoption was the best plan and their own experience of fostering had been influential in their thinking about this. For example, siblings commented:

I remember, we were sat down with the social workers and they said obviously I was too old to be adopted. Well I knew, it wasn't very nice being fostered, you know going to different people all the time. If mum couldn't look after us, and obviously she couldn't, then she [sister] would have had to be fostered.

I went to be fostered and then stayed with my mum and dad for a couple of years and then went back into foster care. We went to another foster place and then to our nana's. Counting up, I've had nine schools and twelve foster carers so I think you should have as few as you can. They've [adopted siblings] had two and that's better.

Other siblings recognised the advantages of adoption saying 'I think he needed long-term stability that adoption gives as opposed to fostering' and 'when you're adopted it's like your parents and when you're fostered it's just somewhere to stop – I think adoption's better for them'. One adult sibling had been opposed to adoption for her two sisters. Acknowledging that they could not stay in the family home, she wanted them to live with her but said she was told that if she persisted in fighting for residence she might lose contact with her sisters altogether. Although direct post-adoption contact was ongoing, there was no communication between this sibling and her sisters' adoptive parents and contact was problematic for everyone. We consider this case in greater detail in Chapters 8 and 9. By the time of our study, the seven birth siblings who expressed a view said they were now happy about the outcome of their brothers' and sisters' adoptions.

All the birth relatives with whom we were able to discuss adoption said it had worked out well and had proved to be best for the children, including three birth mothers, seven grandparents and one sibling all of whom had initially opposed adoption. We cannot compare the responses of birth relatives in our sub-sample with a matched group not having direct post-adoption contact. However, their comments suggest that their ability to see children's progress and to maintain a sense of family connectedness were important factors, which influenced their satisfaction with adoption outcomes for the children. Accepting that adoption was best for the children represents a cognitive position based on direct evidence of children's well-being. It does not mean that birth relatives were necessarily released from feelings of sadness about separation or that all birth mothers were able to relinquish their social and emotional role as parents. As we have seen and will continue to discuss later, not all contact arrangements were unproblematic for adopters, birth relatives or children. Birth relatives' satisfaction with adoption arguably constitutes one of the necessary, although not sufficient conditions, that contribute to the development of working relationships with adopters and the maintenance of beneficial contact over time.

## Birth relatives' satisfaction with frequency and security of contact arrangements

None of the adoptive parents in our sample wanted to increase the frequency of contact beyond their earlier agreement with the agency and birth relatives. Having said that, however, in at least seven of the twenty-one families in this sub-sample adopters had been willing to increase contact at the request of birth relatives or contact had evolved into more informal arrangements including holidays, overnight stays and more frequent visits. Twelve (29 per cent) birth relatives said they wanted more contact than had been agreed, including three of the four birth mothers who initially opposed adoption (although one finally gave her consent). The fourth birth mother who contested her son's adoption was satisfied with the level of contact, which was arranged on a monthly basis. Two relinquishing birth mothers and two birth fathers were happy about contact arrangements. Only three of the eighteen grandparents were dissatisfied with the frequency of contact and two acknowledged that their geographical distance from the adopters' home made extra visits difficult. Six of the eleven siblings wanted more contact. Of those who were satisfied with its frequency, one adult sibling enjoyed flexible contact with overnight stays and lots of two-way telephone calls and four related siblings felt little closeness with their adopted brother who had been born after they left the family home. As Neil (2002b) notes, and as we have commented, the frequency of contact should reflect its purpose. In our sample, direct contact, which was often supplemented with telephone calls and letters, appeared to maintain (rather than to develop) already established relationships, to provide sources of information and to reassure birth relatives and children about each other's well-being. Contact served as a connection that could be developed and extended in future as the children grew up and were able to make their own decisions about contact arrangements. Those birth mothers and siblings who wanted more contact had experienced close (although not always mutually beneficial) relationships with the children. While accepting that adoption was best for the children, they remained unhappy about their separation and the shift in significant relationships that adoption had brought about.

We noted in Chapter 6 that the vast majority of adoptive parents preferred contact arrangements to rest on informal agreements between themselves and birth families. They rejected the constraints they thought would be imposed by a court order and wanted an unfettered ability to exercise control over contact. Birth relatives were much more likely than adopters to want contact protected by an order and 39 per cent of the thirty-eight birth relatives who answered this question said they would have wanted an order had they known it was possible. Birth relatives' wishes for legal security in respect of contact were not always related to the quality of their relationships with adopters. Many had good relationships and contact arrangements were positive and flexible. However, birth relatives recognised that without an order they had relatively little power to insist on contact while adopters, as they saw it, held all the power to give or withhold something that was very important to them. A birth father, who received a section 8 order (Children Act 1989) for post-adoption contact with his son, said:

> It was very important that I see Alan, not on a long-term basis, but a few times a year. The judge agreed with that because of my bringing Alan up and the bond and for me as well. Well, after all the trials and tribulations I thought I needed something on paper. Going through all that, thirty or forty court appearances, you know, and then saying we agree that you can have contact, that was no good to me, I wanted something in black and white. It was nothing to do with my feelings for the adopters. It was for me and the judge said I'll give you this order and he was really very sympathetic.

One birth grandmother had a good relationship with her grandson's adoptive parents. They had agreed to post-adoption contact before an adoption order was made but the grandmother would have preferred an order 'just in case':

We were told beforehand that the adoption laws had changed and we would be able to see him, I think that helped knowing that. I don't know how I would have felt if I had never seen him again. We agreed twice a year but we go every four to six weeks. The adopters got it sorted out and they said 'come any time you want, just give us a ring when you want to see him'. But a court order – in a way it would be a bit of security, it would just give you a bit of security.

Of the fourteen birth relatives who would have preferred an order for contact, we could identify only six where this attitude reflected problematic issues associated with adoption and/or contact or continuing fears about loss. In two situations contact involved, first, the birth grandmother, mother and adult sister from the same family who were all having direct monthly contact and, second, another adult birth sister who was having direct contact with her two adopted siblings. All these birth relatives had initially been opposed to adoption and in both of these families (kinship networks) contact was problematic for birth-family members, adopters and children. Because of these difficulties readers will find references to these two kinship networks in other chapters as we explore adoption and contact from the standpoint of individuals who are located on different sides of the adoption triangle. One birth mother who initially opposed adoption, but finally gave her agreement, was afraid that contact might stop without an order, and one birth sibling who was looked after by the local authority was similarly anxious about losing contact with his sisters. Of course we cannot speak for those birth relatives whom we were unable to interview, but it is perhaps noteworthy that well over half of birth-family members in our sub-sample were content to leave contact arrangements to trust. They might have answered differently if we had asked this question prior to adoption. However, at the very least their responses suggest that trust and security had grown from their experience of contact and adopters' willingness to keep their promises.

## Special Guardianship: an alternative to adoption?

Section 115 of the Adoption and Children Act 2002 amends the Children Act 1989 to introduce special guardianship orders. Very few adoptive parents felt that special guardianship would provide sufficient security, control and mutual belonging for themselves and for the children who were growing up in their families. We asked birth relatives what they thought about this legal arrangement for providing permanent placements without extinguishing birth parents' parental responsibility or severing children's legal connection with their birth families. We had expected that special guardianship would present an appealing option somewhere between children remaining in local-authority care and birth families losing their legal status through adoption. It was surprising to find that from the perspective of birth relatives, special guardianship was thought to introduce as many problems as it might solve. Only one maternal grandmother, one birth mother and one sibling said they would have preferred special guardianship to adoption. These were the birth relatives referred to above who had also opposed adoption and who expressed the wish for a contact order. Seven birth relatives were very cautious about special guardianship and felt that its appropriateness would depend on birth parents' attitudes and their willingness to co-operate with children's guardians. The remaining twenty-eight birth relatives who answered this question rejected special guardianship for similar reasons to the adoptive parents in our sample. They felt it was insecure for the children and prone to disturbance by birth parents who were unhappy about their children growing up elsewhere. Their comments are exemplified as follows:

> I don't actually think that would have worked. With adoption, it's sort of, it's finalised and it's easy for people to understand what their roles and responsibilities are within the arrangements. We were lucky to have contact but if I'd been too close, if I'd been the mother, it would have been too difficult to be involved after they'd actually gone. I don't think you can do that, I don't think it's fair on the children.
>
> (Maternal aunt)

> Well, no, I don't think that would work because it's putting a spanner in the works. To me it's like you've still got a part in that lad's life. I would feel like he's really on loan or on lease and I don't like it that way.
>
> (Birth father)

> I don't think that would work. For instance, if I started saying that I thought Sean should change schools because I had a parental right I think it would cause havoc. I think there'd be slanging matches all round. It could be like a tug of war with the child.
>
> (Contesting birth mother)

> I just don't think it's right. How can a parent get a bond with a child if she feels that another mum has those rights. The parents have to bond with the child, not the natural mother. Bonding with a child is not just about loving them, it's protecting them and giving them all that you can and doing it in the way you think is right. You have either got the child and it's yours or they belong to somebody else and they're never yours. I'm thinking about his adoptive mum taking this child on knowing she could do whatever was in his best interests, change his name, which they did. He is part of their family, not my family.
>
> (Relinquishing birth mother)

## Direct contact: personal comfort, role comfort and satisfaction

In Chapter 6 we considered issues associated with adopters' personal and parental comfort and satisfaction with contact. We think this is also a useful conceptual framework to analyse and explain birth relatives' perceptions, although we have changed an assessment of adopters' *parental comfort* to birth relatives' expressions of *role comfort* to reflect the latter group's different relationships with the children. As might be expected, all the birth relatives with whom we discussed contact could identify their satisfaction in terms of advantages for themselves. Some birth relatives also described advantages for other participants in contact arrangements. However, rather like the adopters, birth relatives' perceptions of advantages flowing from contact were not always accompanied by feelings of personal comfort or comfort with their changed role in the children's lives. The most commonly articulated advantage of contact was that it enabled birth relatives to see the children growing up and to gain reassurance that they were well and happy. All the birth mothers and fathers gave this as the only or most important advantage of direct contact. The four birth mothers who were initially opposed to adoption also felt that contact made their children happy and served to confirm their continuing emotional significance for the children. The two relinquishing birth mothers of children with Down's syndrome were unsure about whether their children benefited from contact. Fifteen of the eighteen grandparents also emphasised the importance of seeing how their grandchildren were getting on while the others simply said they wanted contact because they loved the children. Having first-hand evidence of the children's well-being was also important for aunts and an uncle, while this was identified by six of the eleven birth siblings as the major advantage of contact. They said, for example:

It helps me in the sense that I know he's all right and I like to know who he looks like in the family and who he's taking after and about his school. And every time you see him, they change don't they as they grow older, and it's marvellous the change, you know, you watch them each step. I like to know he's all right.

(Birth mother initially opposed to adoption but who eventually gave her consent)

It helps me knowing they're safe, they're enjoying life, generally I just love the way they're living. Because it's a way of life I could never have given them. It's not because they're rich or anything like that, it's just living life how it should be lived.

(Birth father)

It's good getting a cuddle from him and seeing he's happy. He's getting to understand why he was adopted. He knows he's never short of love.

(Maternal grandfather)

The best thing is to see him growing up, how he's progressing and getting on in life. We like the idea of him knowing about his mum and that he has met his brother and sister. He knows who his grandparents and the rest of his family are.

(Maternal grandmother)

Other birth relatives said 'I get to see her growing up and, it's hard to explain, I just am her grandma and I get to see her' and 'it's contact with a blood-family member, knowing they have a sister who loves them'.

Birth relatives were most likely to describe advantages for the children in terms of their relationship and the children's pleasure in seeing them. Seventeen (45 per cent) of the thirty-eight birth relatives who responded to this question went further than this. They explained that they thought contact helped the children by providing access to family histories and information, contributing to their sense of identity and confirming that their birth families still loved and cared about them. A maternal aunt reflects this thinking in her comments:

> I think we felt at the start that they'd had enough difficulties and problems in their lives without sort of cutting off the people who'd loved them and looked after them, they didn't need that. So now they've got a granddad and an aunt who can love them and look after them and help them out with things. They've got other family as well obviously but it did seem pointless to deprive them of people who'd actually tried to look after them and I think in the future obviously it will be good for them to have some information about their background so it's not cut off completely. If they need anything, if they need to know things, they'll come and ask me, won't they?
>
> (Maternal aunt)

We also asked birth relatives whether they thought contact had any advantages for adoptive parents. While all birth relatives could identify advantages for themselves and nearly half thought contact had specific benefits for the children, only six mentioned any gains for adoptive parents. Two grandparents cited the provision of information as helpful to adopters, and a grandparent and two aunts said that if contact made the children happy this would also benefit their adoptive parents. One aunt thought that contact would demonstrate birth relatives' permission for the adopters to assume a parenting role. The adopters in our sample had attended preparation groups where it was emphasised that contact would be in the best interests of their children. As we have explained, they were willing to maintain contact for as long as they felt it was advantageous for the children and/or short-term parental discomfort was outweighed by the anticipation of long-term benefits. Although some birth relatives identified contact as benefiting children in specific ways, it was evident that their own needs for reassurance, family continuity and emotional gratification were uppermost in their minds. These motivational factors coincided in most cases with children's needs and wishes and with adopters' perceptions of the advantages that flowed from contact. In a small number of cases, however, birth relatives appeared to be so caught up with their own needs that this caused discomfort for the children and/or adoptive parents. This serves as a reminder that birth families also require help to deal with their feelings about adoption, separation and loss. They, as much as adopters, need preparation and support for managing contact visits and understanding and accepting the purpose of direct contact (Mason and Selman 1997 and 1998; Crank 2002).

When considering personal comfort expressed by birth relatives, we are concerned with the extent to which they felt satisfied and relaxed about contact arrangements and at ease during visits. Role comfort refers to birth relatives' accommodation of children's new (adoptive) family relationships and their feelings about the social and emotional 'space' that they occupy in the children's lives. While Howe (1996: 5) refers to the 'ever more complex demands made on adopters', similar observations might equally be made about birth relatives who are involved in direct post-adoption contact. Neil (2002b: 15) points out that 'a key psychological issue for birth relatives after adoption is to adjust to their changed role in the child's life, the reality that their child is also part of another family'. This reality is likely to be acutely experienced during direct contact when birth relatives are visitors to the adoptive home, when they witness parent–child relationships acted out between children and their adoptive parents, and when children talk about their (adoptive) extended families and their everyday activities. Birth relatives only get an occasional glimpse of the children's new and often very different lives. We might not be surprised, therefore, if birth relatives felt some discomfort about their role and relationships with the children during contact. Table 7.1 summarises our assessment of birth relatives' personal and role comfort in the context of direct contact.

Most birth relatives felt comfortable about contact arrangements, accepted their changed role and were relaxed and happy during meetings with the children. For some this rewarding state of affairs had taken time and perseverance and, as we have seen, this was particularly so for the two relinquishing birth mothers. Grandparents, aunts and siblings did not experience role discomfort, feeling that the children still related to them in ways that confirmed their (birth) familial status and emotional significance. They said things like:

> If it's nice we might go to the park, have a walk or something like that. When we're inside we might watch a video or read him a book. He sits on my knee. When we walk in he shouts 'it's granddad and grandma' and then straight for the toffee bag and then he jumps on top of you.
>
> (Maternal grandfather)

*Table 7.1* Birth relatives' personal and role comfort in relation to direct contact

| Birth relatives with contact | Personal and role comfort both *satisfactory* | Personal comfort problematic, role comfort satisfactory | Personal comfort satisfactory, role comfort problematic | Personal and role comfort both problematic |
|---|---|---|---|---|
| Mothers | 3 | 0 | 3 | 0 |
| Fathers | 2 | 0 | 0 | 0 |
| Grandparents | 17 | 0 | 0 | 1 |
| Aunts/Uncle | 5 | 0 | 0 | 0 |
| Siblings | 6 | 0 | 4 | 1 |
| Total | 33 | 0 | 7 | 2 |

When they come here, it's just as if it's never stopped. You'd have to see the boys when they come here. Immediately they grab hold of you, they kiss you, they hug you, this is the way they are. And everyone's quite easy. When we pick the boys up they fly to you straight away. There's no fresh contact, it's just as though it's ongoing. Put it this way, it's not a matter of access, we are just out and out grandparents, that's all it is.

(Maternal grandfather)

They don't remember mum and dad but they do remember me and our brother. It's mainly me they remember most because when they were little I used to look after them a lot and they remember me as their big brother who was really nice to them and that's how they still see me.

(Sibling)

If the adopters had been awkward it might have been different but we feel part of each other's family. Their other adopted daughter regards us as her aunts and uncle now. Our niece has got extra aunts and uncles – she has three families instead of two.

(Maternal aunt)

The four related birth siblings who felt a degree of role discomfort did so because they had never lived with their adopted brother and felt they lacked a sibling relationship with him. They struggled to describe their feelings towards him but said they were different from how they felt about each other. He was more like a friend whom they saw from time to time, they did not quite know how to relate to him during contact and they did not think about him between visits. We have already met the adult birth sister who expressed both personal and role discomfort. She opposed adoption for her two sisters, was blamed by her mother for seeking residence and felt rejected by her sisters' adoptive parents with whom she had no contact. Her sense of personal discomfort arose from her mother's insistence that she should pass messages and presents to the girls and attempt to persuade them to see her. She felt pushed out of her sisters' everyday lives and expressed a sense of alienation from her own family and her sisters' adoptive family. This sibling's role discomfort was related to her perception that her sisters' adoptive parents refused to acknowledge her familial status or her emotional significance. Personal and role discomfort for the only grandparent arose for particular reasons. The local authority placed her grandchild with this grandmother but she was unable to cope with his behaviour and felt she had rejected him. She said:

When he talks and smiles I wonder how I could have done what I did and I have a big guilt trip about putting him back in care. He doesn't make a lot of eye contact with me unless I speak to him and then he answers me. But each time is a little bit easier and helping me to get over what happened and my guilt. The more I see him, the better it gets. I wouldn't have liked not to see him – he is my grandson after all. I just feel sad because of what happened. It was my fault.

(Maternal grandmother)

Three birth mothers felt relaxed and comfortable during contact visits and their personal comfort was not an issue. However, we assessed them as suffering from role discomfort during contact. Two had opposed adoption and one finally agreed at the 'eleventh hour'. They confirmed that they thought of themselves as their children's mothers and had difficulty accommodating the adopters' parenting role. They felt unhappy when the children referred to their adopters as mum and dad and looked for indications of some continuing emotional attachment from their children. We were able to talk to the children of these birth mothers and, as we will see in Chapter 8, they all expressed problematic feelings in relation to contact and/or adoption. While the children all said they were happy with their adoptive parents, some significant emotional issues remained unresolved for the children and their birth mothers.

## Conclusion: birth relatives and direct post-adoption contact

It is heartening to see that birth relatives were reassured by the way adoption had worked out for the children. Unfortunately we cannot say how far these birth relatives reflected the views and experiences of those we were unable to interview. For this sub-sample, however, it seems clear that the majority of birth relatives were enjoying what they saw as beneficial contact, which was accompanied by personal and role comfort. Only nine of forty-two birth relatives suffered problems associated with personal and/or role discomfort in relation to contact. These nine relatives came from six families and in three cases their discomfort was matched by adoptive parents' feelings. In the other three families, one involving a grandmother and the other two birth mothers, the adoptive parents did not describe any discomfort about contact. What does emerge from our interviews with birth relatives is the way in which adults had to work at developing relationships, respecting each other's roles and allowing each other social and emotional 'space' which appropriately reflected their familial relationships with the children. We were struck again by an apparent lack of preparation or support to help birth relatives accomplish these tasks and by the way individuals were thrown back on their own resources to work things out as they went along. Many birth relatives were pleased and relieved to see social services withdrawing from their lives. Help with managing their feelings about adoption and contact, understanding their role and the purpose of contact for children and responding to difficulties or disruptions in contact arrangements might be most effectively provided by services that were not involved in the initial adoption planning. Early discussions and accessible mediation and support are clearly important to all the adults who are involved in post-adoption contact.

## Summary

- This chapter considers interviews with birth relatives having direct contact with the children. These include six birth mothers, two fathers, eighteen grandparents, five aunts, an uncle and eleven birth siblings who were not adopted by families in our sample.

- Three birth mothers, seven grandparents and one of the seven siblings who expressed a view were initially opposed to adoption. One further birth mother remained opposed to adoption for many months before giving her agreement. By the time of the study all birth relatives were satisfied that adoption was best for the children.

- Twelve (29 per cent) of birth relatives would have liked more frequent contact and fourteen (37 per cent) of the thirty-eight birth relatives answering this question would have preferred an order protecting contact rather than relying on informal arrangements.

- Only three birth relatives of the thirty-eight answering this question thought that special guardianship was preferable to adoption. Birth relatives identified insecurity for the children and disruption by birth parents as weighing against special guardianship where children needed to grow up with substitute families.

- The vast majority of birth relatives felt that the most important advantage of direct contact was their ability to see the children growing up and to obtain reassurance that they were well and happy.

- Nine birth relatives from six families experienced personal and/or role discomfort in relation to contact and/or adoption. Three of these were birth mothers who found it difficult to relinquish their parenting role and were upset by the parent–child relationship between their children and their adoptive parents.

# 8 Children's thoughts and feelings

## Adoption and post-adoption contact

### Introduction: the children

In Chapter 4 we described the characteristics of ninety-six children who had been adopted by the sixty-one families in our sample where continuing direct contact with their birth relatives had been arranged. Fifty-one of these children agreed to talk to us about their experience of adoption and contact, of whom forty-three also completed 'clouds'. A further eight children agreed to express their thoughts by filling in the 'clouds' although they declined an interview. This chapter is primarily concerned with the thoughts and feelings of these fifty-nine children, although in our detailed consideration of sibling contact we also discuss the feelings of eleven non-adopted birth siblings who talked to us about their contact with some of the study children. Thomas *et al.* (1999: 138) comment about their work with adopted children, 'when talking about contact, some of the children expressed feelings of sadness, loss and loneliness'. This reflects our research experience but, as we will see, many more children described happy situations where they felt safe and loved in their adoptive families and valued the opportunity to spend time with their birth relatives. It is possible that non-respondents share features that are relevant to an investigation. Researchers must therefore be wary about drawing conclusions that may only be valid for the group of respondents in a particular sub-sample. Our knowledge of the children's circumstances and reasons for non-participation in the research interviews suggest that any bias introduced by non-respondents is likely to be minimal. Only nine children refused to talk to us and the adoptive parents of a further four did not want them to be interviewed. One child's adoption had recently been disrupted but contact was not identified as a significant reason for the family's difficulties.

Of the children in this sub-sample very few (14 per cent) were aged 6 or 7. We had not intended to interview such young children but they insisted on talking to us! Twenty-seven (46 per cent) children were between 8 and 10 years old and nineteen children (32 per cent) were between 11 and 13. Five children were aged over 13 years. Most of these children and young people could talk about adoption and contact with considerable experience. Only six of them had lived with their adoptive families for less than three years, thirty-two (54 per cent) had been placed for between three and five years and twenty-one (36 per cent) were well-established members of their families, having lived with them for longer than five years. We spoke to eight children in three families where contact stopped on adoption although it was initially planned to continue. As might be expected from our analysis in Chapter 4, the vast majority of children in the sub-sample had been placed with their adoptive families for reasons associated with neglectful and/or abusive parenting. Only four children had been accommodated under section 20 of the Children Act 1989 prior to placement for adoption; in three cases their mother had died and one child's mother, who could not 'bond' with her, requested adoption. Their care histories left these children with a legacy of instability. Only one child moved straight from her birth to her adoptive family because the foster carers, with whom she was initially placed, decided to adopt her. Three children experienced only one intermediary placement between birth parents and adopters but twenty-four (41 per cent) had two or three 'in-care' placements and a further twenty-five (42 per cent) children experienced more than three placements before joining their adoptive families. Information was not available for six children. Table 8.1 identifies birth relatives with whom post-adoption contact was agreed for children in this sub-sample.

Analysis of children's comments is complicated when they have contact with several birth relatives because they rarely differentiate between specific individuals. This usually means that children's feelings about contact are consistent towards all the birth relatives who are involved. We point out where it is apparent that children experience contact with individuals in a more or less comfortable and satisfying way. In Chapter 4, we also noted issues associated with trying to engage children as participants in research and we must add a word of caution here. Our approach was open ended, tentative, exploratory and, as far as possible, without any hint of prior expectations that might influence children's answers. However, our focus was on adoption and contact and, while we accept children's accounts as valid expressions of their thoughts and feelings at the time, it must be

*Table 8.1* Birth relatives for whom contact was agreed with children in the sub-sample

| Birth relatives with whom direct contact agreed | Number of children in sub-sample | Number of adoptive families in sub-sample |
|---|---|---|
| Birth mothers only | 4 | 2 |
| Birth fathers only | 3 | 2 |
| Birth mothers and others, including grandparent(s) and/or siblings | 12 | 7 |
| Birth father, paternal grandmother and aunt | 3 | 1 |
| Grandparents only | 6 | 4 |
| Grandparents and others, including siblings and an aunt | 7 | 3 |
| Aunts/uncle only | 1 | 1 |
| Siblings only | 23 | 15 |
| Total | 59 | 35 |

acknowledged that they may feel differently when they are not being invited to concentrate on these particular issues.

## Children and adoption

The 'clouds' invited children to complete the question 'the difference between adoption and fostering is . . . ' and children who we interviewed were also asked if they could tell us about the difference. Forty-seven (80 per cent) children identified relevant differences between adoption and fostering in reasonably clear terms. For thirty-six children the major distinction related to the permanence of adoption, while eleven children expressed ideas associated with getting a new Mum and Dad and the significance of going to court. Children impressed us with their evident relief that their new families were 'forever'. For example:

> With adoption you have the home you're in for as long as you want it to be your home and with fostering you have to move houses a lot.
>
> (Elizabeth, aged 11)

> The foster people look after you and then give you away.
>
> (Ruth, aged 9)

> With fostering you are staying with different people and with adoption you live with your new Mum and Dad forever.
>
> (June, aged 12)

> You are with people who love you and not people who are keeping you for a short time and who end up getting rid of you.
>
> (Jasmine, aged 12)

We wanted to identify how children and young people felt about being adopted. This was discussed during interviews and via the 'clouds', which asked children to complete the sentence 'being adopted makes me feel . . .'. Fifty-three (90 per cent) children unequivocally indicated that they were happy about adoption and relationships in their adoptive families. Two major themes characterised children's responses in this context. First, there was a strong theme relating to permanence and security. Children were happy because they had a Mum and Dad and a family from which they did not anticipate having to move. Second, and this is perhaps unsurprising given children's histories of neglect and abuse, they said they were happy because they felt safe and loved. Children explained:

> I'm happy. This is because I know that I am safe and nothing bad is going to happen. Also, I feel really happy because I know that people really do love me and care for me and I don't have to move around anymore.
>
> (Charlotte, aged 12)

I wanted our own Mum and Dad like other children. You can see your real Mum and you can see your adoptive Mum and Dad – actually, I love them [adopters] to bits.

(Ben, aged 11)

I wanted someone – you know – to love me and I wanted to stay in one place.

(Penny, aged 14)

Other children simply commented that adoption made them feel 'happy', 'great', 'safe and loved', 'safe and secure', 'happy – enjoying it', 'wanted and happy' and so on. Of the six children who expressed some equivocation about adoption, three children reported they felt 'happy and sad' at the same time, one said adoption made her curious about what had happened in the past and one child said adoption felt 'like no-one wanted me when I was a baby'. One child avoided answering this question. There were seven children who, although describing themselves as happy in their adoptive families, also expressed distress or ambivalence about the decision to place them for adoption and the loss of their birth families. These children were able to articulate difficult and complex feelings in response to loss and separation. Martin was 10 years old, had been with his adoptive family for four years and had direct contact with his birth mother. He said that if given the choice he would prefer to live with his birth mother. At the same time, however, he expressed himself as being 'really extremely happy' about adoption and his adoptive family. Ann, aged 12, had been living with her adoptive family for five years and, together with her adopted sibling, continued to see her birth mother. She said about adoption that she was upset about leaving her Mum and:

If I'm naughty or something and like I'm crying and I have to go up to my bedroom then I always think of her [Lucy, the birth mum] and memories of her. I still think of her and the happy times that we'd had. I didn't really want to move because I didn't want to live with anyone else, I wanted to live with Lucy. I really didn't understand why I had to move away. When I see her I mostly talk about being with her – I say 'oh I really, really want to be with you'. I know [adoptive] Mum and Dad love me now and I know Lucy wants me to be with her . . . and I know at the end of the day I can just . . . I know that Sue and Thomas [adoptive parents] are going to be there and I know that Lucy is going to be there for me.

Ann commented about contact with her birth mother:

Yes, it's great, I love it, I love going to see Lucy. I miss her a lot. Oh, I'm just determined to get there. I want to see her.

In Martin and Ann's situations we were able to talk to the children, their adoptive parents and their birth mothers and these 'triangles' are discussed at greater length in Chapter 9. However, during our interviews these birth mothers expressed resistance to relinquishing their parental role to adoptive parents. Both said they anticipated their children would come back to live with them when they were old enough to make their own decisions. It seems likely that the children's conflicting feelings were, to at least some extent, encouraged by contact with their birth mothers. Martin said 'she [birth mother] asks me about school and says that she misses me – I feel sad'. His birth mother reported saying to Martin 'just because you live with them doesn't mean I don't love you – I'll always love you'. She continued 'he's always said he's coming home and I said when you're old enough'. Ann's mother described them as having a very, very close bond and said 'I still think I am their mother and nothing will ever change that'. In Chapter 6, we did not identify contact arrangements in these two cases as problematic according to adoptive parents' levels of comfort or satisfaction. Despite children's and birth mothers' attitudes, adoptive parents felt no significant discomfort and thought contact was in the children's best interests. This may be related to the fact that, as Martin and Ann reported, they felt strong attachments to their adoptive families as well as to their birth mothers and their birth mothers could also identify benefits flowing from adoption. Additionally, the adults managed their feelings and relationships in such a way that they were able to maintain contact without generating significant interpersonal conflict. We also suggested in Chapter 6 that, where adopters experienced contact as comfortable and advantageous for their children, it was likely to be beneficial or at least not damaging for the children. It might be thought that, in the light of Martin and Ann's experience, we should revise this observation. However, it is unlikely that depriving the children of contact with their birth mothers would have been beneficial in terms of easing their sadness and allowing them to attach unequivocally to their adoptive parents. Complete severance may have increased their distress. Both children wanted as much contact with their birth mothers as they could get.

Of the remaining five children who expressed mixed feelings about adoption, three were having indirect contact and two were not having any form of contact with birth parents. Lindy, aged 9, was adopted with her two siblings and had lived with her adoptive family for five years. While it was originally intended that direct contact with her mother and maternal grandmother should continue post-adoption, arrangements were stopped on adoption because contact was not considered to be in the children's best interests. Indirect contact was substituted for direct contact. Lindy told us she wanted to live with her birth mother. However, at the same time she said 'I'm happy here' and, in relation to her adoptive parents and birth mother, she commented 'I love all of them'. She continued:

> I don't know where Margaret's [birth mother] gone. I'm bothered, I'm bothered about seeing Margaret. I think about her very much, I think about her every night. I'd like to see her. I want to carry on seeing Margaret – it's not fair.

Ruth had been living with her adoptive family for nearly three years, was 9 years old and had direct contact with her maternal grandparents. She said about her adoption:

> When I first came here I knew I was going to be happy because they said nice things like they wanted me, so I stayed here and I want to stay here forever. I like them very much and that's why I want to stay here.

She added, however, 'I want to go to [birth] Mum and Dad – I'll go there for a little while and then I'll come and visit here again'. Ruth was 'very sad' that she could not see her birth parents and siblings who were living at home. Sheila was 12, placed with her adoptive family for eight years and having direct contact with her adopted sibling and indirect contact with birth parents. She said she loved her adoptive parents but intended to live with her birth parents when she was older:

> I'll go and see my old Mum and Dad and tell them I want to live with you again or they might live with me. Adoption is not so good – I'd like to see my real parents, they were good to me.

Gerry, aged 12, had lived in his adoptive family for eleven years. He was placed with his sibling and they had direct contact with four further siblings and indirect contact with birth parents. He said of his adoptive family 'it's nice here – my Mum's lovely'. When we offered him a wish, Gerry responded:

> I wish I wasn't born into a family that couldn't look after me and I didn't have to go through the process of fostering and adoption and I could be brought up from a baby by the people who gave birth to me.

Together with her sister, Tracy, aged 9, had lived in her adoptive home for nearly four years. The girls had direct contact with their older brother and indirect contact with their birth mother. Although Tracy refused to talk to us, she completed the 'clouds'. She conveyed her feelings about adoption as being 'happy because I know I will be with a good family'. However, in response to the prompt 'what I would like to happen when I'm older is . . .' she said 'for all the real family to get back together'. The adopters were well aware of the girls' sadness about separation from their birth mother and reported that the children would tell them about their feelings. Tracy's adoptive father said, 'the little one, Tracy, would say "I'm going back to Mummy"'. While the adopters felt the children's grief had been apparent for about a year and had diminished as they became more settled, Tracy still seemed to harbour a desire for reunion with her birth family.

For some children, adoption seems to be experienced as a 'mixed blessing'. Many adoptive parents were aware that their children had strong attachments to birth parents but we were left with the impression that these children kept their sadness and distress largely to themselves. It was in the private sphere of thoughts and feelings that children managed the tension between affection for their adoptive parents and a sense of loss for their birth families.

## Terminating contact: children's wishes and feelings

Continuing contact with at least one birth parent was arranged for eight children in three families but was terminated on adoption because it was subsequently assessed as damaging for the children. In the discussion above we refer to Lindy's distress about termination of contact with her birth mother. Lindy's 7-year-old sister expressed a similar sense of loss. She too was happy about her adoption and said 'it's smashing, I like it with Mum and Dad and it's a good thing we've got a new Mummy and Daddy'. She added:

> I'd like to see what she [birth mother] looks like. I can't actually remember – I'm sad we don't see her – we never see her. I feel sad I can't see Margaret any more.

Children in two families experienced contact more negatively and, despite professional expectations about its continuation, they eventually managed to convey their unhappiness with the arrangements. The adoptive parents of siblings, Melody (10), Emma (9) and Henry (8) explained their growing awareness that the children were distressed by contact with their birth parents:

> It became obvious they were extremely frightened of her [birth mother] and they weren't themselves. They were saying and doing things to please her, which they didn't really want to. This two-year period – it wasn't until the end of this when Melody plucked up the courage to say 'I don't want to go' and then Emma saying 'well, I don't really want to go but I think I ought to'. It had taken them a two-year period to feel safe enough here, confident enough to say 'we don't want it, we have never wanted it'. A lot of their body language was telling me. It got to the stage where the children were saying 'don't leave us here, we don't want to be here on our own'. Then the guardian *ad litem* came and the children made it clear they wanted no contact with their birth mother. Eventually the message got through but I was made to feel that I wasn't an expert in this matter.
>
> (Adoptive mother)

The children told us how they had felt about contact. Melody said:

> Well it was upsetting really because they weren't saying very nice things to us. They were saying they were disagreeing with my [adoptive] Mum and Dad and she [birth mother] was just disagreeing all the time. My Dad wasn't as bad – my other Dad – because he didn't really disagree that much. It's just that we said to our Mum and Dad we didn't want to see them all the time. I told the social worker. I was more happy then because I didn't have to keep seeing them.

Emma echoed Melody's feelings:

> Well, when I kept going to visit she kept whispering things saying 'aren't you going to get your hair long' because it was really, really short. She said she was going to get us high boots, she promised us but she hasn't. I didn't really want to see her. I was really scared to tell people I didn't want to see them because I thought they wouldn't take any notice and would just keep taking us there. And the other social workers we had didn't take any notice of us. Then the new social worker [guardian *ad litem*] asked us 'do you want to go and see them anymore' and we said 'no' and she arranged that.

Henry described contact with his birth mother as follows:

> Every time we went she gave us a present to make us think she was our real, very real Mum and she wanted us to come back to her, that's why. But I wanted to stay with my [adoptive] Mum.

Henry said that contact with his birth parents was OK 'as long as they didn't nick us'.

George (9) and his sibling Lilly (7) had lived with their adoptive parents for two years. The children had not seen their birth father for at least two years prior to their placement for adoption. When social services located their father, contact was reinstated at fortnightly intervals with the intention that its frequency should be reviewed and adjusted as necessary. Initially the adopters handed the children over to their father at a neutral venue and he was allowed to take them away for several hours. The children were so distressed about this arrangement that the adopters subsequently invited the birth father to collect them from home. After several months Lilly refused to leave the house with her father. George's adoptive mother described his distress about contact:

> I think it was Thursday morning and George should have been going on Sunday to see him. He was getting ready for school and he started to cry and we couldn't get out of him what the problem was so we had to ring up school and say he wouldn't be coming in. It took us about four hours for him to say he didn't want to go to his father and the only reason he had been going was because he thought he had to go. And with that I rang the social worker up and put George on the phone . . . He was very angry, he showed a lot of temper, we had like fits of temper. It was like an anger thing basically because in their own minds I think they were being made to do something they didn't want to do.

George said, accompanied by Lilly nodding in agreement:

> I'll tell you something my Mum and Dad do, why I like Mum and Dad because they're always nice to me . . . I like Mum and Dad a lot – at night we give

them a kiss and a hug before I go to sleep. We didn't want to see our other Dad because we hate him. He wanted his own little children not us. Our old Dad hated us a lot and he had about ten women, didn't he? We're happy to be adopted and we don't want to see him.

Although we did not invite children to divulge any fears about contact with birth parents, two children spontaneously expressed very strong feelings in this context. We describe them here because we were struck by the way in which private fears and destructive images served to erode these children's sense of well-being. Emma (9) is one of a sibling group of three to which we have referred above, where the children tried to tell social workers they did not want to see their birth parents. Although contact with her birth mother had been terminated at least a year before our research, Emma was still very fearful:

> I do love my Mum and Dad that I've got. I want to have a happy family but I didn't like my old family – well, sometimes I think about them – I have nightmares about them. Well, sometimes it's that Alex [birth mother] is going to come and take us away and then there is something about killing my Mum and Dad. And my other worry is because I don't want Alex to know where we live. If I saw her I would hold on to my Mum's hand tightly. I think, you know, I'm scared really that she (adoptive mother) might meet Alex. We don't know where they (birth parents) live but they might live near. And she might go to my Mum's office and work there and my Mum might not notice and then she might, when everybody's gone, she might stab my Mum and then might go near and do something else which I really, really don't want to happen.

The adoptive parents understood that Emma was afraid of her birth mother but we wonder whether they appreciated the depth of her fearful and troubled thoughts. Although Jane (16) had been living with her adoptive family for six years, she retained strong feelings about her birth parents. She said:

> I don't like her. I don't want her to know our address – she'd put the windows through – she's done it once. No, not after what she did to me. She locked me up and gave me no food so I nearly died. We all kept getting bashed. My Dad whipped us on our arms. It upsets me when I talk about it, it won't go away. She keeps threatening everyone and I don't want her turning up at our school. I want to see my sister but I don't want to see my birth Mum and I'm glad my Dad has died. He kept hitting us and leaving us locked in while he went to the pub.

Jane's adoptive parents seemed unaware that her history continued to evoke such strong feelings. There may have been other children who experienced similarly powerful emotions but who chose not to share them with us. Emma and Jane, and the other children to whom we have referred above, serve as a reminder that children are not simply vessels into which we can pour good experiences and relationships to displace those that have been painful or problematic. Children and young people have their own subjectivities, which are not always transparent to the significant adults in their lives. The majority of children in this sub-sample gave every indication that they were happy, settled and relatively carefree. Practitioners and carers must, however, be sensitive to the possibility that some children struggle privately with intense feelings. These may require specific acknowledgement and focused intervention to help children shed the burden of anxiety, grief and anger.

## Direct contact: children's perceptions of comfort and satisfaction

Macaskill (2002) reports on children's experience of direct contact with adult birth relatives. From information provided by adopters, foster carers, social workers and children she concludes that 12 per cent of children experienced contact positively, 57 per cent responded both positively and negatively, 6 per cent were neutral and for 25 per cent of children contact was 'very negative'. Rushton *et al.* (2001) found that the carers of children in adoptive and permanent foster families viewed *sibling* contact as positive for the majority of children. Sibling contact was reported as negative for 14 per cent of singly placed children and for 21 per cent of jointly placed children. The children in our sub-sample told us how they felt about direct contact with their birth relatives. As we did for adoptive parents, we have analysed children's responses in relation to their comfort about contact visits and their satisfaction with contact arrangements. By using the term satisfaction here, we are referring to children's perceptions about the relative advantages of contact and their wishes about its continuation. While some children experienced discomfort associated with meeting birth relatives, they could also perceive benefits that encouraged them to want contact. Table 8.2 identifies children's expressed feelings of comfort and satisfaction in response to contact with different members of their birth families.

Although it may look from Table 8.2 as if there are six additional children to the 59 included in our sub-sample, this is because six children in four families had contact arrangements falling in the category of birth mother together with other birth relatives. While all six children having direct contact with their birth mothers described comfort, satisfaction or both as problematic, they also reported contact with siblings as being good in both areas. These children therefore appear in two experiential categories to reflect their accounts of contact with different birth relatives. The remaining children expressed consistent feelings towards all birth relatives where they were involved in mixed contact arrangements.

Overall the majority of children (78 per cent) expressed comfort and satisfaction, which characterised their contact with *all* birth relatives. Additionally, the six children mentioned above were comfortable and satisfied with sibling contact although they felt very differently about contact with their birth mothers and, in one case, their maternal grandmother. As might be expected, there were no children who felt comfortable but dissatisfied with contact. Five children expressed discomfort

*Table 8.2* Children's reported experience of comfort and satisfaction with direct contact

| Birth relatives with whom children having contact | Children: comfort and satisfaction unproblematic | Children: comfort good but satisfaction problematic | Children: comfort problematic but satisfaction good | Children: comfort and satisfaction both problematic |
|---|---|---|---|---|
| Birth mother only | 4 | 0 | 0 | 0 |
| Birth father only | 1 | 0 | 0 | 2 |
| Birth mothers together with other birth relatives | 12 | 0 | 2 | 4 |
| Birth father, paternal grandmother and aunt | 3 | 0 | 0 | 0 |
| Grandparents only | 5 | 0 | 0 | 1 |
| Grandparents together with other birth relatives | 7 | 0 | 0 | 0 |
| Aunts/uncles only | 1 | 0 | 0 | 0 |
| Siblings only | 19 | 0 | 3 | 1 |
| Total | 52 | 0 | 5 | 8 |

accompanied by satisfaction with contact. One child, Martin, to whom we referred earlier in this chapter, was upset by his birth mother's allusions to loving and missing him. Sean, aged 12, was distressed by the antipathy between his adoptive parents and birth mother, the cross-questioning to which he was subjected by both parties and his birth mother's resistance to accepting his adoption and his life in a different family. He said of his birth mother and grandmother:

> Sometimes they ask me things. They'll ask if I like it here or if I'm happy, and other things like that. I think they're trying to put me off liking my [adoptive] Mum and Dad. Because they're trying to force me not to like my Mum and Dad. If I had a really good time last time, I think it will be another good time this time. If they said things last time then I worry about if they'll say anything again. I came home once crying my eyes out because of all these questions. And when I was there my [birth] Mum said 'do you know this man at the bar – he's your real Dad' – that made me upset.

Sean did not know the 'man at the bar' and remained uncertain about whether he was his birth father. Martin's and Sean's situations and interaction between their adoptive and birth families are discussed in greater detail in Chapter 9. Virginia, aged 8, enjoyed contact with her older sister but was anxious and upset about the uncertainty and unreliability of contact arrangements. As her adoptive parents commented in Chapter 6, Virginia's sister failed to return their telephone calls and they were not always sure where she was living. Virginia worried about losing contact with her sister and was 'sad' that she did not see her more often. Elizabeth (11) and Charlotte (12) are siblings placed in the same adoptive family. They both described discomfort arising from contact with their birth sister who had spent several years 'in care' prior to living with their birth mother. Charlotte's account also covers comments made by Elizabeth:

> I feel a bit nervous 'cos we don't know what she's going to be like. Sometimes she's a bit rough with both of us and like she's gone off with one of us and left one of us out, me – yes it's me – or she does it the opposite way. It's just that she knocks you about and like when she holds your hand she squeezes it and messes around . . . I feel a bit upset – she does as well, she's upset as well – it's hard to say goodbye without getting upset. She thinks it's her fault we're not living together, she says that sometimes. Inside she gets hurt, she used to cry a lot. I worry about her 'cos you don't know what she's going to do, if she's going to run away 'cos she has done before, and whether she's going to come back.

Despite their discomfort, all five children were keen to maintain contact and said they felt sad and disappointed when it was time to say goodbye. Eight children expressed both discomfort and dissatisfaction with contact. Their birth father prompted these feelings in George and Lilly, and Melody, Emma and Henry attributed their attitudes to contact with their birth mother. We discussed the situations and views of these children earlier in this chapter. Ted, aged 9, was distressed by contact with his birth mother and made his own decision not to see her when she failed to initiate contact for a year. Carol (14) was upset by her grandparents' rejection of her adoptive mother, their refusal to see Carol with her adoptive mother present and their excessively critical attitudes. She commented that she did not want to visit her grandparents while they were 'behaving like children'. Jane (16) referred to the discomfort that arose from her birth sister's tendency to exclude her during visits in favour of her jointly adopted sibling. Jane's distress outweighed any benefits of contact and, although she had tentatively renewed contact at the time of the research, this followed four years during which she refused to see her sister. She said contact was:

> Horrible, I thought I wasn't there so I stopped going again. They just totally ignored me. So I thought I wasn't supposed to be there 'cos she [birth sister] wanted Janet instead of me and I thought of walking out but decided I'd better not.

Although the numbers of children are small when grouped according to birth relatives with whom they were having contact, it is evident that children were more likely to feel uncomfortable and dissatisfied about contact with birth parents than was the case for other birth relatives.

## Children's and adoptive parents' perceptions of contact

In Chapter 6 we discussed adoptive parents' reactions to contact in relation to feelings of personal and parental comfort and satisfaction with its advantages for their children. Readers may remember that parental comfort relates to how far adopters felt their children were significantly upset or disturbed by contact. It is interesting to compare adopters' and their children's feelings in the context of parental comfort, children's comfort and their respective assessment of satisfaction. Adoptive parents expressed parental discomfort, and parental discomfort combined with dissatisfaction, in respect of at least one contact arrangement for twenty-four children. We were unable to interview seven of these children. However, when we talked to the remaining seventeen children we found that adoptive parents of twelve children in eight families identified feelings associated with parental discomfort and dissatisfaction that matched those of their children for at least one contact arrangement. Adopters' feelings in two families did not reflect those of their five children. In one family, to which we referred earlier in this chapter and where the children's contact with their birth mother and grandmother had been terminated on adoption, the adopters expressed personal and parental discomfort and dissatisfaction about contact. Their three children, however, did not appear to feel any discomfort with contact and were distressed about its termination. In the other family, adopters felt parental discomfort about contact with a birth sibling but comfort was not an issue for their two children. Additionally, there was one family where the adopted child felt upset during contact with his birth mother, but the adopters did not report parental discomfort. Looked at another way, of the fifty-nine children in this sub-sample, fifty-three (90 per cent) described feelings about contact that were consistent with feelings experienced by their adoptive parents. This consistency includes positive and negative attitudes to contact in terms of children's and adopters' feelings of comfort and satisfaction.

One tentative conclusion we might draw from this finding is that the vast majority of adoptive parents did not express reservations about contact only because *they* found it difficult to accept their children's links with birth relatives. Where adopters did experience contact as problematic, this was more likely to stem from an accurate perception that contact was causing problems for their children. Having said that, however, it is important to remember that we cannot check the match between adopters' and children's feelings about contact for the remaining thirty-seven children in our sample where we were unable to talk to them or to obtain information via the 'clouds'.

## Contact and saying goodbye

Children were much less likely to articulate the advantages arising from contact than were their adoptive parents. They talked instead about how contact made them feel and for most children this was a good feeling. Children said for example:

> It's nice, very happy. I like playing with them, they hug us, it's just a nice feeling.
>
> (Contact with birth father, paternal grandmother and paternal aunt)

> It just makes me feel happy. They're like a real family. It's hard to put into words. I just know they're real family.
>
> (Contact with aunts and uncle)

> It's exciting. When you've had them the whole day you think yes, this is good. Yes I like it because it would make me feel sadder if I didn't see them. I do like to cuddle them 'cos they're really pleased to see us. They always say 'hi' and we run up to them.
>
> (Contact with maternal grandparents)

> It just makes me feel a lot happier. We just tell them that we love them.
>
> (Contact with maternal grandparents and aunt)

Of the forty-eight children who retained direct contact with at least one birth relative and who answered the question, 60 per cent said they would like more frequent contact. The other 40 per cent were happy about contact arrangements. Thirty-eight (64 per cent) of the fifty-nine children said they felt sad or upset when it was time to say goodbye to their birth relatives. However, the majority of children indicated that this feeling was transitory. It was only the small number of children, discussed earlier in this chapter, who were unhappy about separation from their birth families or termination of contact where this sadness became a more prevalent feature of their experience. Seven children expressed relief about the end of contact visits. This group includes all the children who responded to contact with discomfort and dissatisfaction. Nine children felt good about having had contact and five children said they had no particular feelings about ending their meetings with birth relatives.

Children's accounts of their feelings about adoption and contact suggest that, for most of them, their everyday lives were not clouded by a significant sense of loss. However, when we asked them if they ever worried about anything thirty-six (61 per cent) children identified issues associated with adoption or their birth families. Twenty-five children expressed worries about their birth relatives' well-being. They worried about their grandparents dying or being lonely, about the welfare of siblings who were not settled with a family and, where children had seen birth parents dependent on alcohol and drugs, about whether they would hurt themselves. Five children worried about birth relatives finding out where they lived, four were concerned that they might lose contact with birth relatives and two children worried that their adoptions might not work out. Direct contact went some way towards quelling these worries for many children and adoptive parents were aware of its importance in this respect.

## Sibling relationships: placement and contact

We decided to look in some detail at sibling contact because of the particular significance which has been attributed to sibling relationships during childhood and into adulthood (Lamb and Sutton-Smith 1982; Cicirelli 1994). Where a local authority is looking after children, section 23(7) of the Children Act 1989 states that siblings should be placed together 'so far as is reasonably practicable' and consistent with each child's welfare. Policy and practice guidance from the Department of Health (1990, 1998a, 2001d) reinforces the importance of placing siblings in the same accommodation and of maintaining contact between them if this is not possible. In its guidance on the preparation of care plans, the Department of Health (1999) also recommends the inclusion of information about different plans for siblings and arrangements for contact if they are placed separately. Although the Children (Scotland) Act 1995 does not specifically require siblings to be placed together, accompanying guidance makes it clear that joint-placements should be arranged unless this would be contrary to the children's best interests (Scottish Office 1997, paragraph 19). Emphasising the significance of sibling relationships, the Department of Health (2001d) has issued draft guidance on helping adult siblings who have been separated through adoption. It is evident that policy and guidance in the UK stresses the importance of maintaining sibling relationships through joint-placements or continuing contact (Lord and Borthwick 2001: 6). This imperative reflects the widely held view that siblings, especially if they have experienced adversity, tend to develop close and enduring relationships. If contact between siblings is lost this may cause distress or psychological damage. Harrison (1999: 106) suggests, from her study of sibling relationships for long-term looked-after children, that:

> Losing contact with a sibling represented not just the loss of a relationship but also being deprived of a source of information, a potential sense of belonging and, for some young people, an opportunity to continue in a caring role.

However, several factors contribute to the separation of siblings when one or more of them become looked after by local authorities. These include individual decisions about their welfare, placement disruption and the availability of appropriate placements. Children also become separated from each other when birth family circumstances lead siblings to enter care at different times or children remain with birth families while their siblings are in care or adopted (Wedge and Mantle 1991; Bilson and Barker 1992/3; Kosonen 1996). Furthermore, research indicates that when siblings are separated, a significant number of them also lose contact with each other (Bilson and Barker (1992/3; Harrison 1999; Masson *et al.* 1999; Neil 1999; Rushton *et al.* 2001). Some children grow up without any sibling contact and others may lose already established relationships. Our research concentrates on siblings where arrangements were made for the continuation of direct post-adoption contact. We did not set out to identify those siblings with whom contact was lost following the study children's admission to care or their adoption placements. Of the ninety-six children in our overall sample, fifty-seven (59 per cent) were placed with at least one sibling in twenty-five adoptive families. Thirty-nine children were placed singly, although five of them developed sibling relationships with unrelated children who were also adopted by the same family. Apart from these five socially constructed sibling relationships, all the siblings in our study and those with whom they were having direct contact were related by birth. Children's attitudes to their siblings appeared to be unaffected by whether they shared the same birth mother and father or, as in many cases, the same mother only. Direct contact with siblings together with other birth relatives was agreed for twenty-five children in seventeen families. Families in our sample had adopted eight siblings in this group for whom contact was agreed. Thirty-two children in twenty families had contact arrangements with siblings only. Eleven of these children visited siblings who were also adopted by families in our sample. The remaining thirty-nine children were subject to contact arrangements with birth relatives other than siblings. Seven of the study children with sibling contact arrangements had lost contact with one or more siblings since their adoption. However, at the time of the research a further eight children were having contact with siblings who were not originally included in contact agreements.

Contact involving siblings was agreed for thirty-four (58 per cent) of the fifty-nine children in the sub-sample. For twenty-three of these children contact was arranged with siblings only, while eleven children had contact agreements with siblings plus other birth relatives. Nine of these thirty-four children had contact arrangements with siblings also included in the sub-sample as they had all been adopted *within* our sample of sixty-one families. Three children in the sub-sample had lost contact with their siblings since arrangements were agreed. In addition to specifically discussing sibling contact with thirty-four children in the sub-sample we were able to talk to eleven birth siblings who had direct contact with our study children and who were either still 'in care' or living independently.

## Sibling contact: children's wishes and feelings

As we noted earlier, thirty-three of the thirty-four children in the sub-sample for whom sibling contact had been agreed, expressed satisfaction with contact and wanted it to continue. Only three of these children described discomfort in association with sibling contact. Maureen, aged 20, was not included in our study sample. She had been adopted by one of the sample families and wanted to talk to us about separation from her birth family. We include Maureen here because she provides an insight into the feelings of children and young adults who lose contact with their siblings. Maureen had entered 'care' when she was a baby and had moved between foster and residential placements until joining her adoptive family when she was 9. While in care Maureen was separated from two older sisters and a brother, but remained placed with her sister Theresa. Following her adoption Maureen lost contact with Theresa, but this had been renewed two years before we spoke to her. Maureen expressed her feelings in this way:

I did want to be adopted because I was sick of being pushed about but on the other hand I didn't want to be away from my sister. It sounded better than being pushed around but I would have liked to be with my sister. It didn't bother me about my Mum, I didn't care. Even when they first got in touch with me two years ago I didn't want to see her. My Mum didn't bother me really, my other sisters didn't bother me really. It was only Theresa because we'd been together for so long. I don't regret it [adoption], not one bit. I just wish I could have had my sister Theresa with me. That was the bit that hurt – being separated. When we met again I was happy, I started crying. I just hoped it could be the way it was when we were little. I was living in a bit of a dreamland. I hoped we could all get on and make a fresh start but it didn't work. It's been too long from when I was 9 to nearly 18, just too long. You grow apart, grow different.

Children in the sub-sample varied in the intensity of their feelings for siblings and this appears to be related to the amount of time they had spent together and to the nature of shared experience. For example, Penny (14) was placed with her sister while 'in care' until her sister had to be moved to an alternative placement. Penny said:

I always used to stand up for her. We were best buddies and if anyone ever picked on her I'd always go up to them and give them a battering. I was unhappy when she moved. I used to not eat or anything.

Emma (9) said about contact with her sister:

When I used to see her and she used to come to us, I used to cry because I didn't want her to go. Now, well I miss her but there's no need to cry because she will come and see us again – she's never going to go away. She doesn't cry. Before, I thought she wasn't going to come again, but now I know.

Maggie (9) said:

I'm excited when I'm going to see her because I haven't seen her for ages and I like to go and see my sister – she's a special sister. She's good to me and kind. I'm upset when it's time to go 'cos I like staying with my sister all the time.

Shared history and experiences were also significant in influencing the feelings of birth siblings with whom the study children were having contact. Julia is several years older than her sister, but they were fostered together before the latter was placed for adoption with one of our study families. Julia had this to say about adoption and contact:

I think probably it [adoption] was the best plan. It was maybe a shock for me and I don't know, you always think you'll be together – it was hard. It's nice

– it's obviously nicer than if I didn't see her. I'm learning to know who she is as she's growing up. She's not just my baby sister, she's her own personality and I know she's happy there. It's lovely but when she's gone it's hard then. It's strange. It's just this strange feeling. It's hard when she's gone. For a good week or two afterwards, you know, she's always on my mind and you just, you feel kind of empty. It's weird. You know after a while you settle.

David (16) tried to look after his three younger siblings while they were at home and had finally alerted social services to their abusive situation. The three children were adopted by one of our study families and David maintained direct contact with them. He said:

I'm relaxed because I know they're not with my father and I know they're with a family that does care about them. Well, I see they are well and I know they are happy. It gives me the satisfaction of knowing they are still all right. They're family. I just like their company. I like being with them because they're my family.

Sandy (16) also cared for his two younger sisters who were in our sub-sample and with whom he continued to have direct contact. He said simply: 'I miss my sisters. I'd like to see them every day, I'd like to be with them.'

Some children in our sub-sample had more tenuous links with their siblings and, while wanting contact with them, admitted they felt more like friends than members of their family. Harry (13) was maintaining contact with four sisters who were much older than he was and with whom he shared a limited history. He said about contact:

I used to enjoy it but as you get older . . . I like seeing them. I'd like to see them sometimes, but not too often, once every year or so is OK. They've all gone off now and started new lives. I like to know how they're doing in their lives because they're proper sisters and I think it's important.

Charlotte (12) had spent a very short time living with her sister with whom she continued direct contact. She commented:

Well, I still really like her but she doesn't feel like a proper sister if you know what I mean. She feels like a friend 'cos one of my friends I like a bit more than her. It's difficult 'cos you don't really know her as much.

An older birth sibling having contact with one of our sample children made a similar point. In this case the sibling was fostered with three other siblings and they had never lived with the child in our sample who was born following their removal to 'care'. The birth sibling remarked 'because I don't see him very often, it feels different. It's just like going to visit him as a friend.' Another sibling said: 'I don't think about him very much because he doesn't live here. I don't know what he's like really.'

The significance of sibling contact is clearly influenced by children's history and experience. Sibling relationships may change over time as peer relationships become more or less important and as different siblings reach young adulthood and their interests diverge. Nonetheless, the vast majority of children in our sub-sample, and the siblings with whom they were having contact who spoke to us, were all clear that they valued contact and wanted it to continue. Like many contact arrangements to which we have referred, sibling contact may provide not only current pleasure and reassurance but is also an investment for the future when relationships may change, develop and become of enduring importance.

## Conclusion: listening to children and young people

It is encouraging to find, from talking to children and their adoptive parents, that there is a high level of consistency between their respective perceptions of comfort and satisfaction associated with contact. However, as we have seen in this chapter, some children expressed distress about separation from their birth families and lack of contact with birth parents. Other children had been upset by adult expectations that contact should continue when it caused them significant discomfort. Some children experienced fears and worries with which they appeared to cope alone. The legal framework for attending to children's wishes and feelings is firmly in place. Section 22 (4) and (5) of the Children Act 1989 lays a duty on local authorities to ascertain the wishes and feelings of looked-after children, and to give them due consideration, before making any decision that affects them. Section I of the Adoption and Children Act 2002 lays further duties on agencies and courts where they are making decisions relating to a child's adoption. Among other things, they must consider the child's ascertainable wishes and feelings and 'the relationships which the child has with relatives and with any other person in relation to whom the court or agency considers the relationship to be relevant'. Some children in our sub-sample described complex and sometimes conflicting feelings. Helping children to express and deal with these feelings cannot be ensured by a legal imperative but requires sensitivity, trust and engagement between children and significant adults.

We hope this chapter also serves to demonstrate that separated siblings valued contact even if it was sometimes uncomfortable. For some siblings whose experiential and emotional links were more tenuous, contact may represent an investment for the future. It is still the case, as the Department of Health (2002b: 6) observes, that when adoption arrangements are made 'siblings are frequently placed apart'. Making, agreeing and maintaining sibling contact therefore becomes important. Adopters in our sample who wanted to start or to repair lapsed contact arrangements with their children's siblings experienced an uphill struggle to get any social work help. Prospective adopters and birth-family members caring for children also need the kind of preparation and education that alerts them to the importance of sibling contact. We can do little better than to finish this chapter with the comments of a birth sister having contact with one of the children in our sample. She said:

He's family. He's our brother. If I didn't see him I would wonder if he was alright. We know he loves us. When we see him he tells us he's missed us and immediately asks when we will meet again.

## Summary

- This chapter considers the feelings of fifty-nine children with whom we were able to discuss adoption and direct contact and the views of a further eleven birth siblings where direct contact had been agreed with children in the study.
- Forty-seven (80 per cent) children were able to differentiate between adoption and fostering in clear terms, which included reference to the permanent nature of adoption, getting a new Mum and Dad and going to court.
- Fifty-three (90 per cent) children said with no hesitation that they were happy about adoption and they felt safe, secure and loved. Seven children expressed feelings of sadness and loss associated with separation from their birth families and placement for adoption, although saying they still felt attached to their adoptive families.
- For eight children comfort and satisfaction was problematic in relation to contact. Six of these children had contact arrangements with birth parents. In five cases contact had been stopped because the courts did not consider its continuation to be in the children's best interests and one adopted child refused to see his birth mother after a lapse in her contact. One child expressed discomfort and dissatisfaction with grandparent contact and the other with sibling contact. Overall, 78 per cent of children in the sub-sample said they were comfortable and satisfied about contact with all the birth relatives who were involved.
- Of the fifty-nine children in the sub-sample, fifty-three described feelings about contact that were consistent with those expressed by their adoptive parents.
- Sibling contact has been given considerable attention in research, practice and policy literature. There is evidence that many children who become looked after by the state will experience separation from their siblings thus directing attention at arrangements for contact. Thirty-three of the thirty-four children and young people in our sub-sample, who were experiencing sibling contact, expressed satisfaction with contact. Only three of these children reported feelings of discomfort, which were not sufficient to interfere with their satisfaction and wishes that contact should continue.

# 9 Views from the triangles

## Introduction: triangular relationships

Parker (1999: 58) emphasises that those contact arrangements appearing outwardly similar may still have different consequences for individuals. This is because participants experience contact from the standpoint of their own particular histories, relationships and expectations. Additionally, contact arrangements and the way in which they impact on people may change over time and under varying circumstances. Although Parker points out that children's needs should primarily inform any assessment of contact, it is also necessary to consider the repercussions for others who are involved since 'contact, by its very nature, entails the interaction of all the participants'. Although some studies on adoption and openness include interviews with children, most research involving participants' views has been conducted with separate samples of adoptive parents and birth relatives who are not involved in the same family networks. It has thus been impossible to compare the perspectives of adults and children who *share* common contact arrangements and who constitute particular kinship networks. Research has not been designed so that we can understand the repercussions of contact for those individuals who occupy the three sides of a single adoption triangle. The only study we have been able to identify, which compares the experiences of participants sharing contact, is that of Grotevant *et al.* (1999) in the USA. However, their study does not focus specifically on face-to-face contact and only includes accounts from twelve cases of matched birth and adoptive parents. Children's perceptions of contact are not included and we cannot tell how their experiences compare with those of adults in the sample. Grotevant *et al.* (1999: 245) note 'to our knowledge, there is no existing research that has attempted to characterise processes at the adoptive kinship network level using data from all participants'.

This chapter discusses our findings from a sub-sample of eleven 'triangles' where we were able to interview adoptive parents, children and birth relatives who were members of the same kinship networks and who thus shared the same contact arrangements. We were particularly interested in three main issues: how participants experienced shared contact arrangements, to what degree they expressed similar feelings about contact and how far individuals were congruent in their attitudes towards each other and perceptions of their relationships. Overall, we were hoping to identify points at which participants' perspectives of contact agreed or diverged. A focus on issues associated with the convergence or divergence of attitudes, feelings and perceptions may point to factors that facilitate or impede beneficial contact.

## The sub-sample of adoption triangles

The eleven adoption kinship networks in this sub-sample involved eighteen children, including three sibling groups of two and two sibling groups of three. Table 9.1 summarises the children's ages at placement for adoption, their ages at the time of the research and the length of time for which they had lived with their adoptive families. With the exception of three siblings who were placed for adoption after their birth mother's death and one child who was placed because of her mother's severe intellectual impairment, all children in the sub-sample had experienced poor parenting and/or multiple forms of abuse. Table 9.2 summarises the reasons given by social workers for adoption decisions in respect of children in this sub-sample. A total of thirty-six reasons were identified as some social workers cited more than one factor as having influenced adoption planning. Below, we provide brief pen pictures of the children and their contact arrangements.

*Table 9.1* Ages of children at placement, time of the research and length of time in placement

| Ages (years) | At time of placement (number of children) | At time of research (number of children) | Length of time in placement (number of children) |
|---|---|---|---|
| 0  to  2 | 4 | 0 | 0 |
| 3  to  5 | 7 | 0 | 10 |
| 6  to  8 | 5 | 5 | 6 |
| 9  to  11 | 2 | 6 | 2 |
| 12  to  14 | 0 | 5 | 0 |
| 15  to  18 | 0 | 2 | 0 |
| Total | 18 | 18 | 18 |

*Table 9.2* Reasons for adoption decisions

| Reasons for adoption decision | Number of children |
|---|---|
| History of emotional abuse | 11 |
| History of physical abuse | 12 |
| Failure to thrive | 1 |
| History of sexual abuse | 6 |
| Birth mother's mental ill-health or severe intellectual impairment | 3 |
| Birth mother died | 3 |
| Total | 36 |

### *Ann and Lee*

Ann and Lee are birth siblings. They are 12 and 8 years old and have lived together with their adoptive parents for five years. Their birth parents refused to give consent to the agency's freeing application for adoption but did not actively contest the order. They have contact with their birth mother and her new husband twice a year. There is a significant geographical distance between them so contact is arranged by social services and takes place in a neutral venue. The visits last for about two hours with the adoptive parents present.

### *Sean*

Sean is 12 years old and was placed with foster carers at the age of 4. His foster carers adopted him when he was 9. His birth mother actively contested the adoption. Agreed contact arrangements involved Sean visiting his maternal grand-parents, birth mother and siblings once a month for a day at his grandparents' home. Sean's grandparents undertook to supervise contact with other family members. However, Sean's grandfather has since died and his grandmother has abandoned supervision. Sean now visits his mother and sister's homes as he wishes. When his maternal grandfather was alive travel arrangements were shared, but since his death Sean's adoptive parents have assumed responsibility for transporting Sean both ways.

### *Martin*

Martin is 10 years old. He was placed with his adoptive parents when he was 6 and adopted two and a half years later. His birth parents agreed to his adoption but only after refusing to co-operate with the adoption plan for many months. Martin sees his birth mother three or four times a year. Although there is no limit on the length of her visit, his mother usually stays for about an hour. She collects Martin from his adoptive home and takes him out. Martin should also have contact with his adopted brother and his sister who is in foster care. Contact with his siblings has now stopped, apparently because Martin's adoptive parents and his siblings' carers could not agree on mutually convenient arrangements.

### *Jane and Janet*

Jane and Janet are 16 and 18 years old and have been with their adoptive parents since they were 9 and 11 respectively. Their birth mother actively contested their adoptions and their birth father was dead. They now see their adult sister and her children about twice a year at her home, although recently they have met at their grandmother's house. Jane and Janet are now old enough to make their own contact arrangements and can see their sister more often if they wish. Their birth mother lives nearby and pressurises their sister to ask them to see her. Janet is happy with these arrangements. However, Jane refused to see her sister for four years because she felt excluded and isolated during visits and was afraid her birth mother might turn up. At the time of the research Jane had recently renewed contact with her sister. There is no contact or communication between Jane and Janet's sister and their adoptive parents.

### Mark

Mark is 9 years old. He was placed with his adoptive family at the age of 6 and was adopted when he was 8. His birth parents refused their agreement to an order freeing him for adoption but did not contest the agency's application. Mark meets up with his birth mother, maternal grandmother and adopted siblings three times a year in a neutral venue. Additionally, he enjoys an extra three meetings annually with his grandmother, either at her home or his adoptive home. He also has further contact with his adopted siblings, which was arranged for six times a year. However, all the siblings live close by and contact arrangements are flexible. Mark's birth mother has started to increase her contact by visiting her mother's house when Mark is there.

### Ian, Dean and Paul

Ian, Dean and Paul are triplets aged 12. They were placed together with their adoptive family when they were 4 and adopted two years later. Their maternal grandparents requested adoption following their birth mother's death, which left no one with parental responsibility for the boys. The children have contact with their maternal grandfather (their grandmother has since died) and maternal aunt three or four times a year, either at their grandfather's or their adoptive home. Contact arrangements are flexible and, because of the distance involved, their grandfather and aunt usually stay for a few days. The boys have also begun to spend some holidays with their grandfather.

### Linda, Julie and Carol

Linda, Julie and Carol are birth siblings aged 10, 9 and 6 respectively. They were placed at the ages of 7, 6 and 2 and adopted together two years later. Their birth mother initially contested adoption applications. The children's birth father was unmarried and did not have parental responsibility. However, he eventually persuaded the birth mother that adoption was best for the children and she finally agreed. The girls have contact with their birth father, paternal aunt and paternal grandmother once a year. Originally, direct contact was arranged for twice a year. However, given the long distances involved in travelling to meetings and grand-mother's increasing frailty, everyone agreed on a reduction to once a year. The families usually spend a few hours together at a recreational venue.

## *Elaine*

Elaine is 13 years old. When she was 4 she was placed with foster carers, who adopted her when she was 10. Elaine's birth mother had severe mental-health problems and refused her agreement to adoption. Direct contact occurs between Elaine and her half-sister who is a young adult living in her own home. A considerable distance between the two families means that visits take place around four times a year but these often include overnight stays at both homes. Between meetings Elaine and her sister frequently phone each other. Elaine's sister sees their birth mother but Elaine does not feel ready to visit her at present. There is letter contact between Elaine and her birth mother and the adopters are willing to initiate direct contact if and when Elaine expresses a wish for this.

## *Trish and Robert*

Trish and Robert are 7-year-old twins. They were placed with their adoptive parents at the age of 2 and adopted a year later. Their birth parents actively contested the adoptions. Trish and Robert see their maternal grandparents who live a long distance away. Contact is open and flexible, the adopters taking the children to their grandparents' house or vice versa. However, because of the distance meetings effectively occur between four and six times a year.

## *Alan*

Alan is 9 years old, was placed with his adoptive family when he was 4 and adopted two years later. His birth mother, who suffered from severe alcohol dependency, contested the adoption but his birth father supported the plan. Alan's birth father visits him at his adoptive home three times a year.

## *Jenny*

Jenny is 9 years old and was placed with foster carers six days after her birth. Her foster carers adopted her when she was 2. Jenny's birth mother has a severe intellectual impairment and was judged to lack the capacity to make a decision about her daughter's adoption. She remains in residential care and Jenny is very unsure about whether she wants to see her. Jenny has direct contact with a number of maternal aunts and uncles and has been told that she can meet her birth mother when she feels ready. While contact was agreed for three times a year, arrangements are very flexible and special family occasions are enjoyed together at each other's homes.

## Agreement to adoption and the enforcement of contact arrangements

Ryburn (1996) suggests that contact can be successfully maintained between birth parents and children after contested adoptions. However, Parker concludes that parental opposition to adoption may introduce tensions and difficulties into contact arrangements. He argues (1999: 49) 'it seems plausible that opposition to the very idea of adoption will lead to the manipulation of contact in ways which make it difficult to manage and confusing for the child'. We were interested in whether direct post-adoption contact was arranged for birth parents who refused their agreement to adoption and in what ways parental attitudes to adoption influenced the nature of direct contact. Only one husband and wife and one birth mother gave their agreement to adoption for four of the eighteen children in this sub-sample. In these two families, the married birth father and the unmarried birth mother had direct contact arrangements, which were continuing. Of the adoptions contested by birth parents in four families, direct post-adoption contact was arranged for only one child with his birth mother. In this case direct contact was continuing at the time of the research between Sean, his birth mother, maternal grandmother, older sister and other siblings. The relationship between Sean's birth mother and his adoptive parents was problematic and Sean's contact with his mother also caused him some unhappiness as we will explain later. Two contesting birth mothers of three children maintained indirect contact with them and one birth mother of two children had no contact at all. In three families where one or both parents refused their agreement to adoption or freeing orders, but did not contest the applications, two birth mothers maintained direct post-adoption contact and one had indirect contact. Parental opposition to adoption was not a bar to continuing contact but, as we shall see, birth mothers' attitudes were related to comfort and satisfaction with contact for various member of the adoption triangles in which they were involved. At the time of adoption, the birth mother of three children was dead and the birth mother of one child lacked mental capacity. Where birth parents were not included in direct contact, children continued to see other members of their birth families.

As we have noted, some advocates of post-adoption contact think courts should be more proactive by making orders for contact under section 8 of the Children Act 1989. In Chapter 3, we discussed judicial attitudes towards attempting to enforce contact through imposing a contact order alongside an adoption order. Judicial imposition of orders for contact is relatively rare (Murch *et al.* 1993) and nine of the eleven contact arrangements in the sub-sample were agreed voluntarily. Courts made section 8 (Children Act 1989) orders for direct post-adoption contact to Alan's birth father and to one of Jenny's maternal aunts who was her mother's legal guardian. In Chapter 6, we noted that in some cases there was confusion about whether courts had made orders for post-adoption contact. Adopters and birth relatives in the sub-sample appeared to understand the status of contact arrangements apart from Sean's adoptive and birth families where there were different perceptions about the basis for contact. Sean's adoptive father understood the court had not made an order but thought they were constrained by their agreement with the agency:

> No, it [contact order] would have been too inflexible but had they imposed an
> order we would have had to live with it. I'm not sure of the legalities, but I

don't think there is anything we can do about it. I think he does have to have some sort of contact. It was laid down in the adoption agreement that he will have some sort of contact.

Sean's adoptive mother had a slightly different perception of the situation and maintained that contact arrangements were entirely voluntary:

> No, I wouldn't want an order, it's more flexible like this. We would not have liked it if it had been set down that we have to do this, that and the other. If they had said to us you still have got to take him twelve or thirteen times a year we wouldn't have been making that decision, the family wouldn't have been making that decision and it wouldn't have felt like we were a family. It would have felt that we were still being governed by social services.

The maternal grandmother who Sean visits was under the impression that direct contact had been secured by a court order:

> I'm glad we got the order. Well, it's Sean's mum, an order is more on our side. If it was left to them [adopters] they could change their minds.

Sean's birth mother had a different perception and was unaware of her right to apply for leave to seek a contact order if the adopters reneged on their promise to facilitate contact:

> I suppose it would be better if it was written down because they could stop contact at any time and I thought they would have because they were getting upset. If they chose to stop contact I don't think there is anything I could do about it. I can't go back to court.

## Experiencing direct contact

Grotevant *et al.* (1999: 239), in their analysis of twelve adoption kinship networks, identify a process of 'collaboration in relationships' through which adults negotiate and manage their interaction to accommodate direct contact. This process unfolds over time and it is not free from tension and difficulties. Our study found some differences of opinion between adoptive and birth families about satisfaction with frequency of contact and other aspects of contact arrangements. However, the majority of adults managed contact in spite of their sometimes different wishes and expectations, engaging in mutual adjustments, revisions and compromises that Grotevant *et al.* (1999: 239) liken to a successful dance. Birth relatives and adopters in only two of the eleven kinship networks in our sub-sample demonstrated such persistently incongruent attitudes and perceptions that contact was problematic for everyone involved. Jane and Janet and Sean were caught up in these two situations.

Detailed analysis of the interviews suggests that several factors contribute to a beneficial experience of contact for adults and children. These are:

- The willingness and ability of adoptive parents and birth relatives to develop positive feelings towards each other and the emergence of a mutual friendship or satisfying relationship.
- Adopters' perceptions that they are given 'permission' to parent by birth relatives and birth relatives' willingness to assume a different role in relation to the children.
- Good communication between all the parties including adopted children.
- Congruent wishes between the parties about the frequency of contact.
- Mutual concern for the child's well-being.

## The development of relationships: respect and liking

While more birth relatives expressed positive feelings about adoptive parents than vice versa, the adults showed a generally high level of congruence in this area. It was clear, however, that a mutually positive attitude was not always an immediate reaction although it could develop over time. Adopters and birth relatives in our sub-sample described a wide range of feelings towards each other including apprehension, ambivalence, sympathy and gratitude. Adopters' feelings were influenced by their children's reactions to contact, how far birth relatives had harmed or protected their children and birth relatives' willingness to accord them a parenting role. Birth relatives' feelings reflected their attitudes towards adoption, their perception that children were well and happy and their sense that adopters openly acknowledged their continuing importance to the children. Sometimes the 'chemistry' was right and the adults just liked each other despite the way in which they had been brought together. Kinship networks where members were most successful at developing satisfying relationships were those characterised by mutual respect and liking. In seven of the eleven kinship networks, mutual respect and liking were evident in relation to some or all of the adults involved in direct contact. Mutual liking between *all* the adults was apparent in four of these kinship networks. With the exception of one birth father, these four contact arrangements involved children's extended birth families. The following examples illustrate positive relationships between all the adults involved in contact.

Alan's adoptive parents and birth father became good friends:

> To his Dad we are just good friends and that will probably be for a long time. With his Mum I have no feelings whatsoever because she's not the right one for Alan. I love it, seeing them together. Tom [birth father] always gives him a kiss and I get one too.
>
> (Adoptive mother)

> We get on so well and we're very open in the way we talk. I could never do anything to hurt those people because they love Alan so much. I could never

put a spanner in the works. And they know that Alan likes to see me so they make it very pleasant for me as well and we all make it very pleasant for each other and I know all the family. When I go to their house it's like going to my house.

(Birth father)

The adoptive mother of the triplets Ian, Dean and Paul had recently lost her mother and father when the boys were placed with them. Her husband's parents were also dead. The boys' birth grandparents seemed to fill a relational gap and were accepted as members of a new extended family.

It's got to the stage where it's just like a natural family, we're like an extended family. Yes, it's like proper grandparents, oh yeah, he's like my Dad maybe because I didn't have a Mum and a Dad and because Jill had just lost her father and mum. I think that's why it's worked so well. They come over here for holidays, we take them out, we treat them like family. They are part of our family.

(Adoptive father)

We get on very well together, Sheila [birth aunt] and I have a very good relationship. It's like having a younger sister. We are quite close. When her mum died, she was ringing me a few times a week.

(Adoptive mother)

It's like having a sister-in-law, something like that. I don't see them a lot but when we do we get on really well. I have a sister quite a bit older than me and Jill is of a similar age, so it's a similar set-up again. It's like having an older sister.

(Birth aunt)

Well, I think right from the start we were determined not to do anything to interfere, we were just trying to be grandparents, nothing more. And I will say this, Jill has always accepted that we are another mother and father to her. She has accepted us very well and even Sheila, she has accepted her as a sister like. Yes, I feel as if Jill is almost a daughter to me, and her husband is a son-in-law like, that's the way we are. We go there and they come here, it's almost as if we're a complete family.

(Birth grandfather)

Three kinship networks were characterised by respect and liking between *some* adults involved in contact. These were networks which each included contact arrangements with extended birth-family members and birth parents. Good relationships, mutual liking and respect had developed between adoptive parents, grandparents and aunts but relationships between adopters and birth parents were ambivalent.

## The development of relationships: sympathy, acceptance and gratitude

Adopters and birth parents with ambivalent relationships in three kinship networks were largely able to manage contact so as to avoid friction. Adopters' attitudes of sympathy and acceptance and birth parents' feelings of gratitude emerged as important factors in facilitating the development of a working relationship. In the seven kinship networks identified above, all birth relatives expressed gratitude towards the adoptive parents. In the three networks with ambivalent relationships, adoptive parents did not express liking or respect for birth parents but felt some degree of sympathy for them and accepted that contact was important for their children. In a further two kinship networks where contact was with birth mothers only, their feelings of gratitude towards the adopters enabled the development of liking on their part. In one of these networks the adoptive parents felt sympathy for the birth mother but did not like her. The adopters expressed neutral feelings and tolerated contact despite preferring that there should be none. In the other network, the adoptive mother felt sympathy towards the birth mother. She appreciated the birth mother's sense of loss and this seemed to encourage affectionate feelings. The adoptive father, however, was less sympathetic and this may have been because he had little involvement in contact. In the last two cases birth relatives expressed gratitude towards the adoptive parents but this did not facilitate the development of good relationships. The following examples illustrate the complexity of feelings that were managed by adults.

Linda, Julie and Carol were having direct contact with their birth father, paternal grandmother and aunt. Their adoptive parents were aware of their birth father's abusive history but accepted contact with him as 'part of the package'. They expressed positive feelings towards their children's grandmother and aunt who they perceived as having tried to care for the girls when they were at home:

> We were happy to go through with it because we knew the children had been rescued by nan and auntie and therefore had a positive relationship with them. We felt more 'iffy' about contact with [birth father] because of what he had done to the kids but felt if we had contact with nan and auntie we had to have it with him too. It works out OK. We are very fond of auntie and little nan.
>
> (Adoptive mother)

The children's grandmother and aunt felt equally positive and said of the adopters 'they are really lovely people, we couldn't have wished for better'. The adoptive parents did not express positive or negative feelings about the birth father who had abused their children. They did not want to convey a message to their children that they liked him or condoned what he had done. However, they wanted contact visits to be beneficial for everyone and were therefore pleasant to their children's father:

> Jim [birth father] – I wish him well. Auntie and their grandma, they're lovely people, and in that sense we do have to remind ourselves that all of those

stories we've heard about contact where it's described as pretty horrific, in that sense ours is pretty good.

(Adoptive father)

In contrast to the adopters' struggle with their feelings about him, the children's birth father showed no ambivalence about the adoptive parents:

They're, how can I put this, they are two nice people in my life who are tops of the table. They've taken on such a load, that I'm very happy. How they are getting on, how things are working out, that's something I would like to have achieved. But because I can't, I am very happy for those people who've got the chance to do it for me. They're the best thing since sliced bread.

Martin sees his birth mother who tends to be unreliable at keeping to contact arrangements. His adoptive parents initially found the visits, which they regard as a 'moral obligation', rather difficult. However, over time the adopters have come to accept his birth mother and have developed a relationship with her:

But I found it difficult to do at the beginning. I did have this feeling, I am his mother now, and it's difficult when you are trying to establish a relationship with a child at the beginning. It's very dodgy and whenever she came at the beginning she would whisper to him at the door and going over the top, 'I love you Martin'. And it didn't help him, he'd be disturbed and we would be left to deal with it and I'd get resentful thinking, yes, it's all very well going off saying 'I love you Martin, I've always loved you', and then I'm left to deal with this disturbed child. But it's fine now. But she's lovely, we are very fond of her, she's a really sweet girl. She's a bit daft with men. That's her problem, anything to do with men and sex, but she's really quite a sweet girl.

(Adoptive mother)

Martin's birth mother also managed to develop a relationship with his adoptive parents and, despite some feelings of personal discomfort, was able to express her gratitude:

I don't hate them or anything, they've done a really good job with him. But in my eyes they are a lot higher up than me, they're quite posh in my eyes and I feel a bit uncomfortable because of the way they talk, they speak posh. I don't resent them, I feel grateful. I feel a bit jealous that they've got my son, but I wouldn't do anything to upset them. I think they are very open. She's very laid back and she's very understanding, and in a way I think that they respect me because of putting Martin first. I think they do very well for me.

Ann and Lee's adoptive parents felt sorry for their children's birth mother:

I think we feel sorry for her really, you know, she doesn't enjoy the best of health, but I think we feel a bit sorry for her.

(Adoptive father)

> I don't resent the contact, she [birth mother] was very accepting. It would have been very different if she had had a different attitude. I felt very guilty about taking her children. I feel sorry for her having to give them up.
>
> (Adoptive mother)

The children's birth mother expressed a complicated mix of feelings. She felt pleased the adopters loved her children and appreciated their efforts to make her feel comfortable. At the same time, however, she felt awkward about her changed role and relationship with the children:

> I've said many a time they are the perfect couple. They absolutely adore the children and you can tell the way they are treated just how much they have put into the relationship. But I feel really awkward because even though I say Ann's my daughter and I'm her mother, they don't feel like my children because their life is just so different. I don't resent it but I feel really awkward when she calls her [adoptive mother] Mummy and she calls him [adoptive father] Daddy . . . But once I'm there the adopters have always made us feel very relaxed and comfortable.

The development of working relationships between adopters and birth relatives was not always associated with feelings of mutual liking. However, in most cases the adults managed to minimise tensions so that contact could work beneficially for the children in whom they shared a joint interest. This was the case for all but two of the eleven contact arrangements in the sub-sample.

## Permission to parent

Grotevant *et al.* (1999) identify adopters' sense of 'entitlement' to act as a child's parents as an important factor in facilitating contact. Reitz and Watson (1992: 125) define entitlement as adoptive parents feeling they have the 'legal and emotional right to parent their child'. While courts confer legal rights, the perception of an emotional right depends on a process of internal attribution. In those cases where birth relatives accepted adopters as their children's new parents, the adopters expressed a secure sense of 'entitlement' and good relationships were established. The quality of relationships between adopters and birth relatives was also influenced by the latter's perception that adoptive parents were not resentful or restrictive about contact. That is, where adopters were also seen to give permission for birth relatives to have an ongoing role in their children's lives. It is perhaps unsurprising that there was a close relationship between respect, liking and a mutual sense of permission. These factors were clearly evident in seven of the eleven kinship networks, six of which involved contact with extended birth-family members. When contact involved birth mothers a more complex picture emerged and this will be discussed in the next section. The following examples illustrate high levels of 'permission to parent':

## Alan's family

It was Tim who told Alan he had a new Mummy and Daddy. He gave Alan permission to call us Mummy and Daddy. It works for us because he fought through the courts for us and wanted us to adopt Alan.

(Adoptive mother)

He used to call me Dad, and for the first time on my visit he said to his mother, 'oh here's Tim'. So that was good because I thought well he's got to accept his new father and call him father by all means and his mother and call me Tim. I don't mind. He's happy with that and so am I. One thing I had to say to myself was, well, I've got to accept that Alan's got new parents and what I've got to do is bow out a little bit. You see I've got to be careful that I don't get too close to him again, in the respect that I've got to accept that his adopters are his parents now and I've got to let them work his life out. And I know this is all about Alan, but there's me and his adoptive parents as well, we've all got lives to lead. As long as we're all happy and I wouldn't want to do anything without their permission regarding Alan, I wouldn't feel right.

(Birth father)

I think things will stay as they are probably for the rest of Alan's life. I would hate for him to lose contact with daddy Tim and I don't think he will.

(Adoptive father)

## Linda, Julie and Carol's family

Adoption, in my view, they are their parents now. You've got to take a step back and whatever those parents say, they have the children there. This is the final absolution for me because when you give children up for adoption, they are not yours anymore. You have given that right up for the best interests of the children and they are their children from the word go. They are theirs and no one else's. You've got to support the adoptive parents, you've got to have a good relationship and you've got to let them know that you're never going to interfere with whatever they decide whether you like it or not. I think that's what makes it work. They are their parents, you're not anymore, you are extended family members.

(Birth aunt)

I'm very happy for those people who've got the chance to do it for me, that they can be Mummy and Daddy. I'm like a sort of stand in Dad because he's taken on the load that I should have had, and as I say, I'm very grateful for what they're doing.

(Birth father)

The children are more secure now, they've got a new Mum and Dad. I feel very grateful that they're the ones who have got the children. If birth parents started to tell adoptive parents what to do it wouldn't work and would be confusing for the children.

(Birth grandmother)

And for our girls in particular, the most important thing we got permission for when they moved in was that they could change their surname to ours. They left their old surname behind and they had their new life starting and they were very proud to have that name. They felt they really belonged and they wanted the adoption date, they wanted their piece of paper, they wanted to know there was no going back and that no matter how horrible they were, we could not send them back. And they didn't really believe us until we went to get the paper. Because they were – they wanted ownership, total ownership.

(Adoptive mother)

Linda, Julie and Carol's feelings also reflected the sense of permission experienced by adults in this kinship network. For example, Carol (age 6) explained how she felt at the end of contact. She said 'quite sad not to see them – just for a few minutes before I go to the Mummy and Daddy who love me'.

## The status of parenthood: conflict and competition

Permission for adopters to be the children's new parents was most easily granted by extended birth-family members who accepted that birth parents were unable to care for their children. However, three of the four birth mothers with direct contact found it difficult to express unconditional permission. One of these birth mothers had contested her son's adoption, one had refused her agreement and one had refused to consent right up to the adoption hearing when she finally agreed. In three kinship networks, birth and adoptive mothers managed to deal with a potential conflict of motherhood in ways that were not disruptive to contact. Despite this, however, three of the four adoptive mothers said that they would prefer not to have contact with birth mothers. The birth mother who was most unequivocal in expressing parenting permission to the adopters had actually refused her agreement to adoption but came to accept that she was unable to provide her children with adequate care. In this instance the adoptive mother of one child was able to overcome her initial feelings of apprehension when she met the birth mother and realised she did not pose a threat. Mark's adoptive mother said of his birth mother:

She is obviously not judging me. I don't know what she thinks of me but she never seems as if she doesn't like me. She feels free to talk to me, which is quite nice. We're happy to go, well we've agreed to go and see her, but I'm his mother. There's no question about that now. The sort of defining part came when he suddenly started calling her Pam rather than Mummy. But probably, to be honest, I'd prefer her to disappear.

Mark's birth mother said:

> If I couldn't see them I'd be really upset. I get on with my children's adoptive parents and the fact that the children live there doesn't bother me. As long as I can still see them growing up – that will do me.

In two cases where birth mothers found it difficult to express parenting permission, the potential for conflict was diffused as adoptive and birth mothers got to know each other. In these situations, feelings of gratitude, sympathy and acceptance enabled the development of sufficiently positive relationships to maintain contact arrangements. Both birth mothers expressed satisfaction about their children's progress and evident happiness in their adoptive families. At the same time, however, both stated that they remained mothers and hoped their children would come back to them when they were older. Martin's adoptive mother said:

> I knew contact was important. I've done a bit of child psychology as a teacher. But I found it difficult to do myself. I'd have this feeling that I'm his mother now, and it's difficult when you are trying to establish a relationship with a child at the beginning. Yes, it's very silly but it's just the way you are at first, a bit threatened and resentful. You go through all that silliness that you can't bear to come out of your mouth, but it's only human. I never feel like that now. And I also think she [birth mother] had to lay her claim when she came. She had to make it clear that she was his mother, she loved him and always would. It's understandable – she is, isn't she? But I think she has changed over it now, I think she's managed to pull away a bit.

Martin's adoptive parents felt some sympathy towards his birth mother and their increasing confidence as parents enabled them to accommodate contact. At the same time Martin's birth mother appreciated that he was best placed with his adoptive family but could not relinquish her status as his mother. She said:

> Well, this last time I saw him he was a lot closer to me, he was giving me a kiss and a cuddle. He sat on my knee and I said to him 'just because you live here doesn't mean I don't love you'. I said to him, 'I'll always love you'. But he doesn't call me Mum. I'm hoping, I don't know, but I'm hoping he will come back.

A similar accommodation was managed in Ann and Lee's kinship network. Their adoptive mother said:

> I think she [birth mother] is always very positive when she sees them and she sees improvements in them every time. That makes it easier, you know, because you're achieving something for her. I try to be fair, you want to make it alright for her, to let her see them.

The birth mother was grateful for the adopters' contribution to her children's well-being but she was not able to relinquish her role as their mother:

> I think what has helped me to come to terms with it is their happiness. They've got more in life now than I could give them – a lot more. But I don't ever want them to forget who I am. I still class myself as their mother whether Ann sees me that way or she doesn't, I don't know. But I still think I am their mother and nothing will ever change that and I'm hoping that Ann, when she gets older, will come and stay here. That's what I'd like.

In these situations, adoptive and birth mothers managed to accommodate rather than to resolve the potential conflict associated with their respective claims to motherhood. Additionally, adopters felt strongly that their status as legal parents provided an important source of security. This helped them manage any emotional tensions arising from contact (Smith and Logan 2002). However, Ann and Martin from the two kinship networks above were very sad about separation from their birth mothers and both expressed a wish to live with them. So, while it appeared that the adults in these kinship networks had reached some form of accommodation, the children reflected their birth mothers' ambivalence about adoption and parenthood. Crank (2002: 109) suggests that workers who are preparing contesting birth parents for post-adoption contact should 'emphasise that they will always be the birth parent and no one can ever change that'. However, Ann and Martin's birth mothers were describing something more than a biological relationship with their children, which encompassed feelings of attachment, emotional closeness and mothering. Readers may remember that we explored Ann and Martin's feelings in Chapter 8. All the other children in the kinship networks discussed above told us they enjoyed meetings with their birth families and wanted them to continue. They were sad when visits came to an end, but for the majority of children this feeling was transitory and was accompanied by confident expectations about further contact.

## Two kinship networks: the failure to develop a working relationship

We noted above that the adults in Sean's and Jane and Jenny's kinship networks had failed to develop a working relationship and contact was problematic for them and for the young people. In both cases there was no evidence of liking, respect or sympathy between the adults and the best that can be said of these situations is that, although they did not like it, the adopters acknowledged the importance of contact for their children.

### Sean's kinship network

Sean's direct-contact arrangements originally included his maternal grandparents, birth mother, older sister and other siblings living with his mother. Contact was every month for a whole day and Sean's grandparents undertook to supervise contact at their house. Initially, Sean's grandfather transported him one way but since his death the adopters have assumed responsibility for both trips. Sean's birth mother was opposed to adoption and contested the application. The contact arrangements were ongoing at the time of the research. From the start, contact was difficult to manage. The adopters felt that monthly visits affected their ability to lead a normal family life. They reported that contact was disruptive for Sean and badly affected his behaviour at home and at school. Contact has been ongoing for eight years. While Sean's adoptive parents would have preferred no or less contact, they had promised to maintain it at the agreed frequency and felt any change might be upsetting for Sean. The adopters had limited contact with Sean's grandmother and none with his birth mother. It was clear the adults did not like each other and none of the factors identified earlier were available to encourage the development of a working relationship. Sean's kinship network was characterised by mutually low permission and competition for parenting status:

> When he first called me Sally I was angry about that. They were pressuring Sean and I explained to him that they were his new Mum and Dad but I was his Mum. They give him a lot but a mother's love you can't replace.
>
> (Birth mother)

> I don't like to think he's got another mother. He used to call her by her Christian name but she stopped him doing that. He now has to call her Mum. Even though we have always thought of him as ours, there's always her presence in the background ready to put the knife in.
>
> (Adoptive mother)

> They've adopted him but they're not his real parents or grandparents. They are quite friendly when they bring him, but I don't think they are overjoyed because I know they don't like his Mum.
>
> (Birth grandmother)

> Apart from the problems it's causing Sean, I'm not interested in them or their problems.
>
> (Adoptive father)

Sean was well aware of the lack of communication and animosity between his adoptive and birth families and he, rather than the adults, had to manage the consequences:

> Sometimes they [birth relatives] ask me things. They'll ask me if I like it here or if I'm happy. I don't really like them asking that because I think they're trying to put me off liking my Mum and Dad. I'd like to ask my birth Mum to stop causing problems because that upsets my adoptive parents and I'd like to ask my adoptive Mum to stop asking me questions. It might do some good if my birth Mum met my adoptive Mum and had a good chat.

In Chapter 8 we discussed Sean's unhappiness, not only about the tensions in his kinship network, but also about some of his birth mother's behaviour. Nonetheless, Sean said he was happy in his adoptive home and intended to maintain contact with his birth family.

### Jane and Janet's kinship network

A combination of factors contributed to tensions for Jane and Janet, their adoptive parents and their adult birth sister with whom they were having contact. Jane and Janet originally had contact with their birth mother as well as their sister, but it was a frightening and disruptive experience and was stopped. Their birth mother blamed their sister for the cessation of contact and asked her to pass on messages to the girls asking them to see her. Jane and Janet were afraid their birth mother might turn up at contact visits. As we saw in Chapter 8, Jane was so distressed about being ignored and excluded during contact that she had stopped visiting her sister and had only recently renewed contact at the time of the research. Jane and Janet's sister expressed a wish to see them more often and longed to be part of their family life. The adoptive parents accepted their daughters' need for contact but were upset when this caused Jane to be unhappy. Crucially, there was no communication between the adopters and Jane and Janet's sister that might allow them to discuss contact arrangements. Incongruent attitudes and expectations and poor communication are illustrated by the following examples:

> It upsets me because Jane comes back, well this last time Jane came back upset. Now that upsets me, so if it's going to upset her I'd rather her not go. I don't really want to say no because I don't really know if she has that little bit of need. But with Jane I think she is waiting for me, all the time waiting for me to say no. Then it takes it out of her hands. I have problems with it. I don't like it.
>
> (Adoptive mother)

> I don't really feel anything for her [birth sister]. I don't know the lady and I wouldn't have any time for her neither. Apparently she wasn't one of the abusers but she was there. I feel she, being the eldest sister, should have helped them.
>
> (Adoptive father)

> I'd like it to be more open. Kim and John [adoptive parents] are like strangers and I would like to know who my sisters are living with and let us all get to know each other. I want open access like ordinary sisters. What happened to them was nothing to do with me but I've lost my sisters. There is a wall there, it's like a brick wall, it's like fighting between us all. If the barriers were down we could be a family.
>
> (Birth sister)

Despite her mother's threatening attitude and her wish to be socially included in the adoptive family, Jane and Janet's sister was unwilling to acknowledge the adoptive mother's parenting role. She said of adoption:

> The proper Mum seems to be written off and not seen as a parent. I don't believe in writing a birth mother off. A mother is a mother and a child deserves a mother.

Janet did not want to see her birth mother but would have liked her sister to visit them in their adoptive home:

> I want to see my sister, I don't want to see my birth Mum again. I don't like her, it just hurts inside when I see her. I'd like my sister to come down here but Mum doesn't like her to come down here. She doesn't want us to have anything to do with the family, it hurts her and my birth Mum might come and make rows again.

In this situation liking, respect and sympathy were absent. Lack of communication and the adopters' ambivalence about contact made it impossible for Jane and Janet's sister to develop a relationship with the adoptive family. The background influence of the girls' birth mother also created additional tension.

## The frequency of contact and changes over time

Openness in adoption must be regarded as a dynamic process, which develops as the needs and circumstances of individuals change over time (Logan 1996; Grotevant and McRoy 1998; Lowe *et al.* 1999; Neil 2002b). What is 'right' for one party in the adoption triangle at any point in time may not be 'right' for other parties, and as individual needs change this may not be in synchrony with the needs of others. The following comment from an adoptive father illustrates this point:

> Yes, the pattern of contact has changed over time, people and their situations change over time. The original contact was with her other auntie and that seemed to work out pretty well until she got married and then it tailed off. She sees more of her Auntie Margaret now and she complains that her sister doesn't see very much of Jenny now, and the main contact is with Auntie Margaret.

By the time we conducted our study, five of eleven contact arrangements in the sub-sample had changed from original agreements.

We asked participants about their satisfaction with the frequency of contact. Six of the eleven kinship networks were highly congruent with matching levels of satisfaction reported by adoptive parents, birth relatives and children (see Figure 9.1). However, contact arrangements within kinship networks sometimes involved combinations of birth-family members. It is therefore important to distinguish

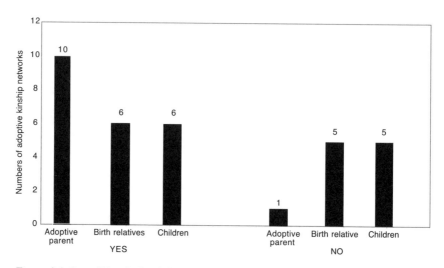

*Figure 9.1* Overall level of satisfaction with contact: kinship networks

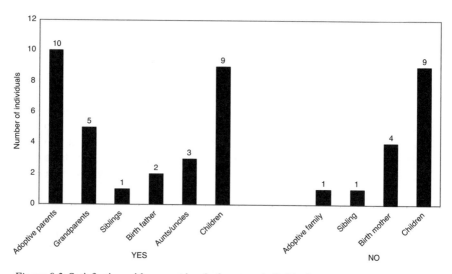

*Figure 9.2* Satisfaction with current level of contact: individuals

between particular birth relatives' satisfaction with frequency and these comparisons are illustrated in Figure 9.2. With the exception of one set of adopters who would have preferred less contact, adoptive parents were satisfied with current arrangements. Overall, there was a relatively high level of congruence between the *adults'* satisfaction with frequency. Apart from one birth sister, all extended birth-family members were happy with current levels of contact, as were the two birth fathers in our sub-sample. In most of these situations, adults were sensitive to each other's needs in terms of control, responsibility for initiating contact and the management of communication.

Five birth relatives wanted more contact, including all four birth mothers and one adult birth sister. Children were the largest group in the sub-sample who said they wanted more frequent contact (see also Macaskill 2002). While nine children placed in six families were happy with the level of contact, the remaining nine in five families said they wanted to see their birth relatives more often. The process of negotiating mutually agreed contact involves adoptive parents, birth relatives and children. However, power is unequally distributed between participants and this asymmetry is likely to affect the outcome (Grotevant *et al.* 1999). This was evident in the cases where birth mothers and children wanted more contact but felt powerless to bring this about. Martin's birth mother wanted to see him more often but felt unable to discuss this with his adopters:

> I didn't like to say really, but I was going to say to her the last time 'can I have him a bit longer?' But I didn't know if it would be the right time or the right thing to do to bring him back here for a couple of hours. I'd like to see him more and for longer, but I didn't like to say. I daren't ask.

Martin's birth mother was nervous about broaching the question of more contact despite his adopters' wish to get things right for her:

> I have to feel that if she wants to see him more she can do so. I think I have to say to her come whenever you want. I can't bear not to do the right thing.
>
> (Adoptive mother)

> We have said she can come whenever she wants to as long as she tells us when she's coming and she can phone whenever she wants.
>
> (Adoptive father)

As we know, Martin said he would live with his birth mother if he had a choice although when asked about adoption he said it made him 'happy – you get loved'.

Mark's birth mother had accepted his adoption. However, she wanted to see him more often and was upset by her mother's more frequent contact arrangements.

> One thing upsets me, my Mum sees Mark more than I do. I see him three times a year and she sees him six times. I'd like to see him more. I'd like him to be back home with me.

Mark's grandmother thought the frequency of contact was about right:

> Three times a year is enough for Pam in my opinion. I think it would upset her if she saw them more often. It would be unsettling for her and Mark. She doesn't like the fact that I go to Mark's home and she doesn't know where he lives or what it's like because she's not allowed to know. She asks why I

won't tell her their address and I tell her I have given my word that I will not disclose it.

Pam found her own way of seeing Mark more often by visiting her mother's house when she knew he was due to have extra contact with his grandmother. The adopters were not resentful or uncomfortable about this. Mark's adoptive mother told us that when she bumped into Pam on one of these unscheduled visits she was surprised to find herself chatting away about ordinary everyday events. She said 'I thought this is unreal – I'm talking to Mark's real mother as if she was just anyone. I wasn't feeling, oh, that's Mark's mother, I was just saying did you get to bed late because you were doing your tapestry?' Mark's adoptive father commented that they were able to accept Pam's extended contact because of the security and 'ownership' conveyed by the adoption order. He said:

> If we were in a situation where you had some level of influence but not the ultimate authority, we wouldn't have taken the same risks and we would have objected to Pam attending contact she shouldn't have done. We would have tended to stick much more rigidly to the letter of an agreement because if you let things run more naturally, you wouldn't know where that was going to lead and if a problem arose you might be unable to sort it out.

Mark said he was happy with his adoptive family but enjoyed seeing his birth family, which he described as 'quite cool'. He said he would like to see his grandmother every weekend.

While some individuals expressed different wishes about the frequency of contact, most arrangements in the sub-sample were working well. Adults who wanted more contact appeared able to accommodate the situation, thus avoiding the introduction of conflict or tension into otherwise acceptable arrangements. Children who wanted more contact seemed able to accept adult decisions and, in this sub-sample at least, did not express anger or frustration about the lack of change. It was evident, however, that some children could anticipate a time when they would not be dependent on the practical assistance of adults to achieve contact. They looked forward to a future when they would be old enough to determine and act upon their own wishes to visit members of their birth families.

## Conclusion: prospects for direct post-adoption contact

In this chapter we have discussed attitudinal and circumstantial factors that facilitated the development and management of relationships in eleven kinship networks. The majority of arrangements were relatively unproblematic and participants experienced direct contact as beneficial. We identified two kinship networks where contact was difficult for children and most adults. The children in these situations wanted contact but were unable to open up communication between adults in their kinship networks. Open and sustained communication between adopters, birth relatives and children inevitably emerged as a central feature in facilitating beneficial contact. Grotevant and McRoy (1998) conclude that openness is an evolutionary process, which is interactively determined by all those involved. In our sub-sample of adoption triangles we were able to see how members of kin-ship networks accommodated, compromised and negotiated contact arrangements over time. Arrangements ran into trouble when this process was hindered by lack of communication and mutual hostility or suspicion. Relationships in kinship networks were easier to manage when contact involved extended birth-family members rather than birth mothers. Figure 9.3 summarises the interaction between attitudinal and affective factors, which influenced the development of beneficial contact for families in our sub-sample of kinship networks.

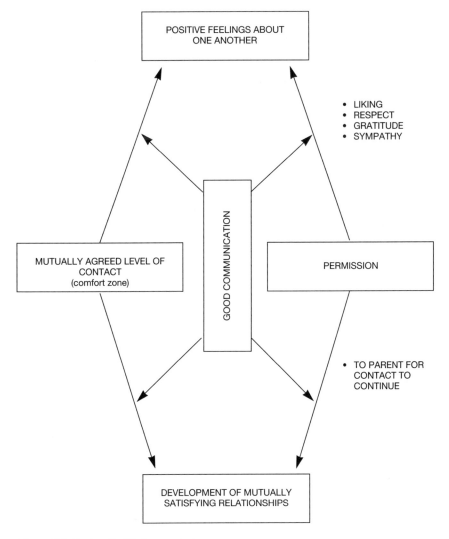

*Figure 9.3* Factors facilitating contact

Historically, critics have been concerned that post-adoption contact and other forms of openness may erode adoptive parents' feelings of 'entitlement' and introduce a sense of insecurity and confusion for children. Findings from this subsample indicate that the legal security of adoption and the way in which adoption acts to construct parenthood can facilitate the development of co-operative relationships within kinship networks. However, relationships that enable contact to be experienced as beneficial require participants to find some common practical and emotional ground on which to work. Social workers can assist this process by preparing adopters, birth relatives and children, helping parties to negotiate and agree contact arrangements and 'rules of engagement' and providing support and mediation if kinship networks encounter serious problems. Finally, we were impressed by the way in which many adopters and birth relatives, with nothing in common apart from the children, could work together to facilitate contact. In order to do this, however, the parties need a clear understanding about the purpose of direct contact (Neil 2002b), their respective kinship roles and the emotional claims that they can legitimately make on children's loyalties and affection. They need, additionally, to be committed to expressing this understanding through their actions and communications. If adults are unable or unwilling to agree about these issues, direct contact is likely to introduce problems for them and, most importantly, for the children.

## Summary

- This chapter has explored the management of contact in eleven kinship networks where we were able to interview adoptive parents, birth relatives and children who shared contact arrangements.
- Between them, the kinship networks included eighteen adopted children and we interviewed four birth mothers, two birth fathers, five maternal grandparents, five aunts and an uncle and three siblings with whom the children were having direct contact.
- Mutual liking and respect between adult members of kinship networks emerged as important for contact to be experienced as beneficial by adults and children. Seven kinship networks were characterised by mutual liking and respect between all or some of the adults involved in contact.
- Even where adults did not like each other, feelings of sympathy, gratitude and acceptance could facilitate the development of a working relationship and beneficial contact.
- Two of the eleven kinship networks lacked the attitudinal and situational factors to enable the development of working relationships and contact was problematic for the adults and children. Communication between birth relatives and adopters was terse or non-existent.
- The majority of adopters and birth relatives were satisfied with the frequency of contact. Adopted children were the largest group who said they wanted more contact.
- Negotiating and managing direct contact was more difficult for adoptive

parents and birth mothers than in situations where other birth relatives were involved. This was particularly the case where birth mothers were unable to relinquish their parenting role to adoptive parents.

# 10 Direct post-adoption contact: benefits, risks and uncertainties

## Sixty-one adoptive families and direct contact

Throughout preceding chapters we have considered direct post-adoption contact from the perspectives of adoptive parents in sixty-one sample families, fifty-nine of their ninety-six children who were able and willing to express their views and forty-two birth relatives who were prepared to talk to us. We have tried to convey the complexity of contact arrangements at the point of agreement between the parties to adoption and as they have changed over time. Additionally, we have attempted to capture and express the nuanced feelings of adopters, children and birth relatives in relation to their experience of adoption and contact. Our study was not designed to evaluate the effects of different contact arrangements according to independent outcome measures for adoptive parents, birth relatives and, most importantly, children. It does not, therefore, meet the requirements of Quinton *et al.* (1997) for longitudinal research that might identify the relationship between specific conditions, varying contact arrangements and particular outcomes for children and adults. However, our respondents' accounts show how relatively simple descriptions of outcome, like comfort and satisfaction with contact, incorporate qualitative and interactive features that influence how far and in what ways participants experience contact as beneficial. For example, we might conclude that personal and parental discomfort with contact indicate negative outcomes for adoptive parents. But, as we explained in Chapter 6, these experiential measures are not related in a straightforward way and are moderated by adopters' attitudes about their children's needs, present and future happiness and the value of long-term benefits over short-term difficulties. We might similarly reach a negative evaluation of contact in the relatively infrequent cases where children and birth relatives expressed discomfort and/or dissatisfaction. However, this conclusion would neglect the way in which other emotional needs supersede feelings of discomfort and motivate children and adults to want contact even if it is experienced as painful and difficult. In our study we have used respondents' accounts, rather than independent outcome measures, to identify how far they experienced contact as beneficial and to explore those features of contact arrangements that influenced their perceptions.

Overall, adoptive parents in forty-one (67 per cent) of our sample families reported that they were comfortable with contact and satisfied it was beneficial for their sixty-five (68 per cent) children. Adopters in a further eleven families expressed personal and/or parental discomfort but retained a belief that contact was best for their children. Thus, parents in fifty-two adoptive families (85 per cent) could identify advantages for themselves and/or their children associated with direct contact. Even if contact caused them some personal or parental discomfort, they believed it would be beneficial for their children in the long term. At the time of the study, the vast majority of these families were continuing contact with birth relatives who were originally included in contact arrangements. All the children except one were still enjoying meetings with at least one birth relative with whom contact had originally been agreed. In one family the adopters expressed personal and parental discomfort about their son's contact with his birth mother but said they thought it would benefit him in the longer term. However, after a long delay in contact from his birth mother, their son refused to see her. Indirect contact was being maintained at the time of the study. There were nine families with fifteen adopted children where adopters expressed dissatisfaction with contact, in association with personal and/or parental discomfort, for at least one contact arrangement involving their children. While it was intended that direct post-adoption contact should continue for these children, it was terminated on adoption for eight children in three adoptive families. Six children in two families lost contact with their birth mothers (three of these children retained contact with a sibling) and two children in a further family lost contact with their birth father. Post-adoption meetings with his birth mother stopped for a further child and his adoptive family when his mother failed to get in touch with the adopters to arrange her visits. In the remaining five families where adopters were dissatisfied with contact, all the children had ongoing meetings with birth relatives who were included in original contact arrangements. We were able to talk to the children in six of these nine families where adopters experienced contact as particularly problematic. The children in five families independently expressed problems relating to comfort and/or satisfaction, which reflected the feelings of their adoptive parents. Three children in one family were distressed that contact with their birth mother had been terminated on adoption, although their adoptive parents were clearly relieved about this.

Fifty-nine children from our sample families were able and willing to convey their feelings about adoption and contact, fifty-one through interviews and eight via completion of the 'clouds'. Seventy-eight per cent of these children experienced contact with all their birth relatives as comfortable and beneficial. While five children identified comfort as an issue, they all wanted contact to continue. Eight children found contact problematic in terms of comfort and satisfaction and six of them expressed relief that direct contact had come to an end. Two young people in this group remained ambivalent about contact and, although they had withdrawn from contact at various times, it was continuing when we conducted the study. Of the fifty-nine children in this sub-sample, we can thus identify only six (10 per cent) who, at the time they talked to us, were so unhappy about contact that they would not have wanted it to continue. Satisfaction with contact was not an issue for any of the forty-two birth relatives who talked to us. They all identified benefits from contact, most usually in terms of seeing that the children were happy and well, maintaining a family connection and wanting children to know that they were still loved and remembered. Over time, birth relatives had come to accept that adoption had turned out to be best for the children, even when they had initially opposed the plan. Nine birth relatives experienced personal and/or role comfort as problematic in connection with contact. Adopters and/or children also expressed issues associated with comfort and satisfaction in response to contact with three birth mothers and five siblings in this group.

## Contact: factors relating to comfort, satisfaction and beneficial experiences

As we noted above, there were only nine families in which adopters found direct contact really problematic in terms of discomfort *and* their assessment that it had no advantages or was damaging for their children. Most of the children from these families, with whom we were able to discuss contact, also experienced meetings with their birth relatives as problematic in relation to comfort and satisfaction. We would love to present readers with a neat package identifying common factors that characterised these kinship networks and which might alert professionals to potential difficulties when they are considering future contact arrangements. For example, birth relatives' opposition to adoption might be expected to impact negatively on adopters' feelings of comfort and satisfaction (Parker 1999) and five of these nine situations included contact with birth relatives who were hostile to adoption. While accepting that adoption was best for the children, they had remained resentful and angry about social-services intervention and their loss of (legal) familial status. However, the remaining four sets of adopters related their feelings to other factors such the frequency of contact, their children's distress, feelings about sharing their children with birth families and the way in which they perceived direct contact as having been demanded and imposed by agencies and birth families.

Additionally, adoptive parents in nineteen families who had direct contact with sixteen birth mothers expressed *satisfaction* about contact, although six of them also felt personal and/or parental discomfort. Of these, eight adoptive families had coped with a birth mother's refusal to agree to adoption or contested adoption proceedings. So, initial parental opposition to adoption is not invariably followed by a problematic experience of contact or adopters' dissatisfaction with its advantages for their children. It is also a mistake to assume that parental agreement to an adoption order constitutes a positive indication of beneficial contact. We found several situations where birth mothers finally agreed to adoption because they caved in under pressure or simply became worn out with the fight. Their formal agreement did not mean they had emotionally relinquished their children or accepted their changed legal and familial role in their children's lives. There is a tendency to concentrate on birth parents' attitudes in relation to decisions about contact but, as we have seen, grandparents and siblings may also feel angry about adoption, separation and the loss of a protective and familial role. The difference between adopters' and children's experience of satisfaction and dissatisfaction with contact was influenced to some extent by birth relatives, and particularly birth mothers' attitudes to adoption, but many other factors were influential. These include qualitative features such as adopters' and birth relatives' natural and learned attitudes of sympathy and openness, their feelings of security about themselves as individuals and parents, their ability to separate their own needs from those of their children and sometimes the almost indefinable impact of personal chemistry. For example, one adoptive mother said, with evident surprise about her children's birth mother who contested their adoptions:

> It's something we had to do in the beginning and it's something that's turned out right. If you can see it's doing your kids good, just go with the flow. I get on great with her [birth mother] – I care about her. I tried very hard in the beginning not to like her because I thought it was the thing to do. I said to my husband 'there must be something wrong with me – I like her'. And he said 'but you don't like people with bleached blonde hair'. And I said 'well, I don't know, I like her, I can't help it'.

Another adoptive mother, who had previously fostered her son, clearly articulated the relationship between her own parental feelings and her son's need to maintain contact with his birth mother:

> I've got full parental control – he's mine. He's settled down. He was less naughty after the adoption because I was secure. I said to him 'you're mine now and it's up to me and you're staying here and you'll be here forever.[9] I think it helped him. But I just knew it was important for him to see his [birth] mother. He used to worry about her when he didn't see her. I suppose I did consider her feelings a bit because she needed to see him, but he needed to see her more. He didn't ask to be taken away from her. He used to say he'd go home to his Mum and visit me in the summer – yes, it hurt but I could see it from his point of view.

The qualities referred to above were in short supply for some birth relatives because of their own experiences and personal difficulties. This is why we should also avoid the assumption that sibling contact is relatively unproblematic. As we discussed in previous chapters, sibling contact was frequently difficult for adopters and children in relation to comfort and satisfaction. Many birth siblings either remained looked after by local authorities or had shared the neglectful and/or abusive parenting experienced by children in our sample. They were not good at sharing relationships and were sometimes demanding, rough and socially unskilled. Adopters are not immune from the impact of insecurity and worries about relationships with their children. As we noted in Chapter 6, we could identify two families where birth mothers delayed or stopped contact after adoption and where we think the adopters' attitudes affected birth mothers' willingness and ability to maintain contact.

Adopters' involvement in negotiating and agreeing contact arrangements, including issues associated with planning, frequency, venue and supervision were also related to attitudes about comfort and satisfaction. In Chapter 5, we identified ten adoptive families who felt they had been compelled to accept contact without any involvement in negotiating and agreeing detailed arrangements. Of these, six families expressed dissatisfaction with contact accompanied by personal and/or parental discomfort, at the time of our study. Adopters from a further three families thought contact was beneficial for their children but experienced personal and/or parental discomfort. However, adopters from three families who were dissatisfied with contact did not feel they had been excluded from earlier negotiations. In Chapter 9, we emphasised the importance of time in allowing adopters and birth relatives the opportunity to get to know each other, to develop working relationships and to mutually adjust their attitudes and expectations. We identified those personal and circumstantial features that enabled participants to experience contact as beneficial. Longitudinal research that relates independent outcome measures, such as children's socio-emotional development, to different contact arrangements and other variables may indicate relationships between contact and more or less favourable outcomes at specific points in time. However, it will fall short of helping us to understand, or anticipate, how qualitative attributes of adopters, birth relatives and children interact and contribute to their experience of contact. It may similarly neglect the process through which adults and children manage, accommodate and develop their relationships over the duration of contact with each other.

## Direct contact: risk and uncertainty

There seems little doubt that quantitative research methodologies have come to be seen as the most effective way of evaluating social work practice in terms of identifying the relationship between interventions and outcomes (White 1997). The ascendancy of quantitative research is also related to a central concern with identifying, quantifying and managing risk. Attention to risk, in the sense of a capacity to calculate probable outcomes, operates to reduce uncertainty about the likely consequences of particular actions (Ericson and Haggerty 1997). It thus encourages confidence that major decisions can be based on evidence about risk and can thus be made in a consistent, systematic and rational way (Brubaker 1984: 2). However, Reddy (1996) argues that planning and decision-making are frequently characterised by uncertainty rather than risk. He suggests that we collude in thinking uncertainty can be transformed into a risk analysis through a 'scientific' approach to measurement, categorisation and calculative techniques. Risk analysis can only work on the basis of probabilities. It cannot provide certainty about what will happen in a particular instance and it cannot incorporate motivational elements, such as emotions and passions, which escape measurement or law-like patterns. Parton (1991, 1996a, 1996b, 1997) has been particularly critical of the emphasis on risk in the context of social work. He says (1998: 23):

Most of the risks which social workers are expected to assess or manage are 'virtual' in the sense that they can neither be directly sensed (touched, heard, seen or smelt), nor subjected to scientific evaluation in any quantified or probabilistic sense. They exist (or are constituted) in the theorems, formulae or procedures we draw upon to think about them. As Adams (1995) and Reddy (1996) have suggested, our obsession with scientised, calculative notions of risk have failed to recognise that much of our experience is better characterised as uncertainty.

In our current state of knowledge it is not possible to calculate the long-term effects on children, adopters and birth families of different contact arrangements. We have not yet established the relationship between situational and personal variables and the risk of relatively harmful or beneficial outcomes associated with contact. As we discussed in Chapter 2, studies have often been imprecise about important variables such as type and frequency of contact, they have not used independent outcome measures and they have not compared outcomes for representative samples with different types of contact. Furthermore, research has not evaluated the effects of contact over time as children move into young adulthood. However, we suspect that for two major reasons research will be unable to eradicate uncertainty in decisions about contact. First, as our own research indicates, the way in which participants experience contact derives from unique interactions of attitudes, feelings, expectations and other attributes that are difficult to quantify and categorise. Second, a risk analysis approach to making decisions cannot account for the process through which adults negotiate and accommodate contact as they engage with each other over time. We are not suggesting researchers should abandon the effort to identify 'risk factors' but we should recognise that uncertainty requires acute investigative, analytical, communication and observational skills when making decisions in *individual* cases. An acknowledgement of uncertainty also requires the recognition that deciding about contact arrangements cannot necessarily constitute a single event. Things may not work out as planned and children, adopters and birth families may need further help later on. In keeping with these comments, Mullender suggests (1999: 11) in relation to research methodologies that have been used to investigate sibling relationships:

> It is important to bear all these limitations in mind when drawing on this school of research and also to remember that, struggling even to integrate general trends, *it does not have the capacity to predict anything about any individual child*. Hence even if you start from what appear to be the clearest likelihoods, you will never know whether you are working with one of the rare exceptions to the suggested rule until events themselves unfold . . . With psychological influences currently in the ascendancy in social work, for example through a whole armoury of 'risk assessments', these words of caution may be particularly necessary.
>
> (Original emphasis)

In individual cases, therefore, those who must make decisions about contact should consider predictions of risk, which may be indicated by research findings. However, they must also attend to those qualitative features of human interaction that may not have been captured through research methodologies and which reflect the particular situational, experiential and personal characteristics of children, adopters and birth relatives who are brought together by post-adoption contact.

## Conclusion: managing uncertainty in decisions about direct post-adoption contact

We have referred, throughout our discussion, to other research that extends or supports our own findings. Pulling this all together and remembering our cautionary comments above, the following summary identifies policy and practice issues that require attention in relation to direct post-adoption contact:

- The sense of security, ownership and control afforded to adoptive parents through an adoption order can facilitate, rather than impede, continuing contact. Policy and practice should aim to enhance adopters' confidence in their role as parents while acknowledging and preparing them for the additional tasks that adoptive parenthood brings with it.
- It is clearly a sensible requirement that agencies and courts should consider existing and desirable arrangements for contact at relevant points in the adoption process. However, pressure to promote and enforce contact through the imposition of a section 8 order (Children Act 1989) should be viewed with caution. Adopters in our sample maintained direct contact because they had promised to do so and because they thought it was in the best interests of their children. They did not want legal interference with their parental control over contact. Research suggests that the most effective way to protect contact arrangements is not via legal enforcement, but through work that is carried out with prospective adopters, birth families and children at the time of matching and placement and thereafter if it is needed.
- Preparatory work with prospective adopters must do more than simply attempting to persuade them that children need contact. It must anticipate the kinds of emotional and management issues that we have identified and prepare them for responding to these. Sensitive work with children is necessary to hear and understand their feelings about separation and contact in individual cases. Similarly, work with birth families must look beyond material facts such as birth parents' agreement to adoption. It must consider, with them, their feelings about adapting to a changed familial role and their willingness and ability to relinquish or modify previous expectations and relationships. Although direct contact with birth mothers was more problematic than other arrangements for adopters and children in our sample, it should not be assumed that preparatory work and support are unnecessary when contact is envisaged with other birth-family members. Neither is it appropriate to miss this work with foster carers who are adopting on the basis that they have already experienced contact

with a child's birth family and are expected to be at ease with contact after adoption.

- Practitioners must think more carefully about the purpose of indirect and direct contact following adoption. Our research indicates that direct contact of more than four to six times annually is likely to be problematic. Contact visits at Christmas and birthdays can also introduce tension and competition for socially and emotionally significant space. Contact that is designed to help children integrate memories and information into a developing sense of identity and to provide opportunities for the future does not have to be so frequent that it erodes adoptive families' ability to sustain their own sense of identity.

- Research indicates some confusion among adoptive parents and birth relatives about the basis of contact arrangements. Where social workers help participants to negotiate and agree contact arrangements, they should ensure agreements are recorded, copies of agreements are given to participants and everyone is clear about their mutual responsibilities.

- Adopters are less likely to find contact problematic when they have been fully involved in discussions about the details and purpose of contact arrangements and where they do not feel compelled to accept contact as a condition of placement. This also requires social workers to undertake thorough discussions with birth relatives about their hopes and expectations for the future. Adopters in our sample found it difficult to cope with situations where birth relatives changed their minds about contact, demanded contact as the basis for their agreement to adoption or where 'forgotten' birth relatives entered negotiations at a late stage in the adoption process. Social workers may not be able to anticipate everything that necessitates a re-think of contact arrangements, for example a children's guardian's or a court's different assessment of a child's needs. However, they can ensure that they maintain open, prompt and supportive communication with prospective adopters as events unfold.

- The vast majority of adoptive parents and birth families in our sample were relieved when social workers withdrew from their lives. However, help with contact arrangements and mediation services were hard to access if and when any of the participants to contact felt they needed them. Initial discussions about contact must accept a degree of uncertainty about how individuals, circumstances and relationships may change over time. Post-adoption services should therefore be clearly identified and responsive to requests for help.

- Direct post-adoption contact should not automatically be viewed as the best arrangement for maintaining openness in adoption along a continuum of alternative options. As our study and other research shows, it can work well and be experienced as beneficial by adopters, children and birth families. However, careful work and assessment must be employed to determine the nature of contact best suited to particular individuals and families.

- Policy-makers, practitioners and researchers must remember that birth and adoptive parenting and experiences of separation and loss are likely to prompt the most profound emotional responses from adults and children. This is why we need to understand their feelings about adoption and contact and why social-work practitioners should seek to develop this understanding for individual members of kinship networks. Stancombe and White (1998: 595) argue that helping is 'a practical-moral affair, which cannot be approached as if rational-technical answers existed'. In the context of our discussion, their observation that 'each encounter is a problem for the subject who acts' must resonate with social workers who are struggling to make the best decisions and with adopters, children and birth families who are brought together through direct post-adoption contact.

Much research serves to confirm what observant practitioners already know or suspect. It may clarify and lend weight to the knowledge and experience that reflexive practitioners already use to inform their work. In some cases research may prompt questions and a critical reappraisal of policy and practice. We hope that this account of our own research on adoption and contact will contribute something to these possibilities.

# References

Adams, J. (1995) *Risk*, London: UCL Press.

Adcock, M., Kaniuk, J. and White, R. (1993) *Exploring Openness in Adoption*, Croydon: Significant Publications.

Adoption Law Reform Group (2000) *Reforming Adoption Law in England and Wales*, London: British Agencies for Adoption and Fostering.

Advisory Board on Family Law (2001) *Making Contact Work: the Facilitation of Arrangements for Contact between Children and their Non-residential Parents: and the Enforcement of Court Orders for Contact – A Consultation Paper*, London: Lord Chancellor's Department.

Advisory Board on Family Law (2002) *Making Contact Work: A Report to the Lord Chancellor on the Facilitation of Arrangements for Contact between Children and their Non-residential Parents and the Enforcement of Court Orders for Contact*, London: Lord Chancellor's Department.

Advisory Council on Child Care (1970) *A Guide to Adoption Practice*, London: HMSO.

Alderson, P. (1995) *Listening to Children: Children, Ethics and Social Research*, Basingstoke: Barnardo's.

Association of British Adoption Agencies (1975) *Opening New Doors: Finding Families for Older and Handicapped Children*, London: Association of British Adoption Agencies.

Avery, R. J. (1998) 'Information disclosure and openness in adoption: state policy and empirical evidence', *Children and Youth Services Review* 20, 1/2: 57–85.

Baran, A., Pannor, R. and Sorosky, A. D. (1976) 'Open adoption', *Social Work* 21: 97–100.

Barth, R. and Berry, M. (1988) *Adoption and Disruption: Rates, Risks and Responses*, New York: Aldine DeGruyter.

Barton, C. (2001) 'Adoption and Children Bill 2001 – don't let them out of your sight', *Family Law* 31: 431–436.

Bauman, Z. (1993) *Postmodern Ethics*, Oxford: Blackwell.

Baumann, C. (1999) 'Adoptive fathers and birth fathers: a study of attitudes', *Child and Adolescent Social Work Journal* 15, 5: 373–391.

Belbas, N. F. (1986) *'Staying in Touch: empathy in Open Adoptions'*, *Smith College Studies in Social Work* 57, 3: 184–198.

Bell, M. and Cranshaw, M. (2000) *Preparation and Selection for Adoption: the Users Experience*, paper presented at British Agencies for Adoption and Fostering Research Symposium, November.

Beresford, B. (1997) *Personal Accounts: Including Disabled Children in Research*, London: Social Policy Research Unit.

Berry, M. (1993) 'Adoptive parents' perceptions of, and comfort with open adoption', *Child Welfare* LXXII, 3: 231–253.

Berry, M., Cavazos Dylla, D., Barth, R. P. and Needell, B. (1998) 'The role of open adoption and the adjustment of adopted children and their families', *Children and Youth Services Review* 20, 1: 151–171.

Bilson, A. and Barker, R. (1992/93) 'Siblings of children in care or accommodation: a neglected area of practice', *Practice* 6, 4: 307–318.

Blyth, E. (1999) 'Secrets and lies: barriers to the exchange of genetic origins information following donor assisted conception', *Adoption and Fostering* 23, 1: 49–58.

Bohman, M. and Sigvardson, S. (1990) 'Outcome in adoption: lessons from longitudinal studies' in D. M. Brodzinsky and M. D. Schechter (eds) *The Psychology of Adoption*, New York: Oxford University Press.

Borland, M., Layborn, A., Hill, M. and Brown, J. (1998) *Middle Childhood: the Perspectives of Children and Parents*, London: Jessica Kingsley.

Borland, M., O'Hara, G. and Triseliotis, J. (1991) *Adoption and Fostering: the Outcome of Permanent Family Placements in Two Scottish Local Authorities*, Edinburgh: Scottish Office.

Bouchier, P., Lambert, L. and Triseliotis, J. (1991) *Parting with a Child for Adoption: a Mother's Perspective*, London: British Agencies for Adoption and Fostering.

Bowerbank, M. W. (1970) 'The case committee – what is its future?', *Child Adoption* 59: 35–38.

Bridge, C. (1993) 'Changing the nature of adoption: law reform in England and New Zealand', *Legal Studies* 18, 81–102.

Brodzinsky, D. (1984) 'New perspectives on adoption revelation', *Adoption and Fostering* 8, 2: 27–32.

Brodzinsky, D. M., Schechter, M. D. and Marantz Henig, R. (1992) *Being Adopted: the Lifelong Search for Self*, New York: Anchor Books.

Brubaker, R. (1984) *The Limits of Rationality: an Essay on the Social and Moral Thought of Max Weber*, London: Allen and Unwin.

Butler, I. and Williamson, H. (1994) *Children Speak: Children, Trauma and Social Work*, London: Longman.

Butler-Sloss, E. (1988) *Report of the Inquiry into Child Abuse in Cleveland 1987*, Cm. 412, London: HMSO.

Casey, D. and Gibberd, A. (2001) 'Adoption and contact', *Family Law* 31: 39–43.

Charlton, L., Crank, M., Kansara, K. and Oliver, C. (1998) *Still Screaming*, Manchester: After Adoption.

Christensen, P. H. and James, A. (eds) (2000) *Research with Children: Perspectives and Practices*, London: Falmer Press.

Churchill, S. R., Carlson, B. and Nybell, L. (1979) *No Child is Un-adoptable*, London: Sage.

Cicchiní, M. (1993) *Development of Responsibility: the Experience of Birth Fathers in Adoption*, Perth: Adoption Research and Counselling Service Inc.

Cicirelli, V. (1994) 'The longest bond: the sibling life cycle' in L. L'Abate (ed.) *Handbook of Developmental Psychology and Psychopathology*, New York: John Wiley and Sons.

Clapton, G. (2001) 'Birth fathers' lives after adoption', *Adoption and Fostering* 25, 4: 50–59.

Clapton, G. (2003) *Birth Fathers and Their Adoption Experiences*, London: Jessica Kingsley.

Clothier, F. (1943) 'The psychology of the adopted child', *Mental Hygiene* 27, 2: 222–230.

Craig, M. (1993) *Communication and Recollections about Adoption and Being Adopted: No Big Deal*, unpublished, copy available from Scottish Office.

Crank, M. (2002) 'Managing and valuing contact with contesting birth families' in H. Argent (ed.) *Staying Connected: Managing Contact Arrangements in Adoption*, London: British Agencies for Adoption and Fostering.

Cullen, D. (1994) 'How amenable are contact disputes to judicial resolution?', *Adoption and Fostering* 18, 1: 31–32.

Dalrymple, J. and Hough, J. (1995) *An Exploration of Children's Rights and Advocacy*, Birmingham: Venture Press.

Department of Health (1990) *The Care of Children: Principles and Practice in Regulations and Guidance*, London: HMSO.

Department of Health (1995) *Moving Goalposts: a Study of Post-Adoption Contact in the North of England*, London: Department of Health.

Department of Health (1996a) *Adoption*, CI (96) 4, London: Department of Health.

Department of Health (1996b) *For Children's Sake: an SSI Inspection of Local Authority Adoption Services*, London: Department of Health.

Department of Health (1998a) *Adoption – Achieving the Right Balance*, LAC (98) 20 and CI (99) 6, London: Department of Health.

Department of Health (1998b) *The Government's Response to the Children's Safeguards Review*, London: The Stationery Office.

Department of Health (1999) *Care Plans and Care Proceedings under the Children Act 1989*, LAC (99) 29.

Department of Health (2000) *Adopting Changes: Survey and Inspection of Local Councils' Adoption Services*, London: Department of Health.

Department of Health (2001a) *Social Services Performance Assessment Framework Indicators 2000–2001*, London: Department of Health.

Department of Health (2001b) *National Adoption Standards for England*, London: Department of Health.

Department of Health (2001c) *Donor Information Consultation: Providing Information about Gamete or Embryo Donors*, London: Department of Health.

Department of Health (2001d) *Adopted Adults and Their Siblings: Draft National Adoption Standards for England and Practice Guidance*, London: Department of Health.

Department of Health (2002a) *Children Adopted from Care in England: 2001/2002*, London: Government Statistical Office.

Department of Health (2002b) *Social Services Performance Assessment Framework Indicators 2001–2002*, London: Department of Health.

Department of Health (2002c) *Providing Effective Adoption Support: Issued for Consultation*, London: Department of Health.

Department of Health and Social Security (1984) *Report of the Committee of Inquiry into Human Fertilisation and Embryology*, Cmnd. 9414, London: HMSO.

Department of Health and Welsh Office (1996) *Adoption: a Service for Children*, London: Department of Health.

Deykin, E., Patti, P. and Ryan, J. (1988) 'Fathers of adopted children: a study of the impact of child surrender on birth fathers', *American Journal of Orthopsychiatry*, 58: 240–248.

Dominick, C. (1988) *Early Contact in Adoption, Contact between Birth Mothers and Adoptive Parents at the Time of and After Adoption*, Research Series 10, Wellington, New Zealand: Department of Social Welfare.

Ellison, M. (1958) *The Adopted Child*, London: Victor Gollancz.

Ericson, R. and Haggerty, K. (1997) *Policing the Risk Society*, Oxford: Clarendon Press.

Etter, J. (1993) 'Levels of co-operation and satisfaction in 56 open adoptions', *Child Welfare* LXXII, 3: 257–267.

Fish, A. and Speirs, C. (1990) 'Biological parents choose adoptive parents: the use of profiles in adoption', *Child Welfare* 64, 2: 129–140.

France, E. (1990) *Interdepartmental Review of Adoption Law Background Paper Number One: International Perspectives*, London: Department of Health.

Fratter, J. (1996) *Adoption with Contact: Implications for Policy and Practice*, London: British Agencies for Adoption and Fostering.

Fratter, J., Rowe, J., Sapsford, D. and Thoburn, J. (1991) *Permanent Family Placement: a Decade of Experience*, London: British Agencies for Adoption and Fostering.

Freeman, M. (1997) *The Moral Status of Children*, The Hague: Kluwer Law International.

Freud, S. (1957) 'Family Romances', *Collected Papers Vol. 5.*, London: Hogarth Press.

Giddens, A. (1990) *The Consequences of Modernity*, Cambridge: Polity Press.

Giddens, A. (1991) *Modernity and Self-identity*, Cambridge: Polity Press.

Goldstein, J., Freud, A. and Solnit, A. J. (1973) *Beyond the Best Interests of the Child*, New York: Free Press.

Goldstein, J., Freud, A. and Solnit, A. J. (1980) *Before the Best Interests of the Child*, New York: Burnett Books.

Gonyo, B. and Watson, K. W. (1988) 'Searching in adoption', *Public Welfare*, Winter: 14–22.

Grey, E. (1971) *A Survey of Adoption in Great Britain*, London: HMSO.

Griffith, K. (1991) 'Access to adoption records: the result of changes in New Zealand law' in A. Mullender (ed.) *Open Adoption the Policy and the Practice*, London, British Agencies for Adoption and Fostering.

Gross, H. E. (1993) 'Open adoption: a research-based literature review and new data', *Child Welfare* LXXII, 3: 269–284.

Grotevant, H. D. and McRoy, R. (1998) *Openness in Adoption: Exploring Family Connections*, London: Sage.

Grotevant, H. D., Ross, N. M., Marchel, M. A. and McRoy, R. G. (1999) 'Adaptive behaviour in adopted children: predictors from early risk, collaboration in relationships within the adoptive kinship network and openness arrangements', *Journal of Adolescent Research* 14, 2: 231–247.

Haimes, E. and Timms, N. (1985) *Adoption, Identity and Social Policy*, Aldershot: Gower Publishing Company Limited.

Harrison, C. (1999) 'Children being looked after and their sibling relationships: the experiences of children in the working partnership with 'lost' parents research project', in A. Mullender (ed.) *We Are Family: Sibling Relationships in Placement and Beyond*, London: British Agencies for Adoption and Fostering.

Harris-Short, S. (2001) 'The Adoption and Children Bill – a fast track to failure?', *Child and Family Law Quarterly* 13, 4: 405–430.

Henney, S. M., Onken, S., McRoy, R. and Grotevant, H. (1998) 'Changing agency practices towards openness in adoption', *Adoption Quarterly* 1, 3: 45–76.

Hill, M. (1997) 'Participatory research with children', *Child and Family Social Work* 2: 171–183.

Hill, M., Lambert, L. and Triseliotis. J. (1989) *Achieving Adoption in Love and Money*, London: National Children's Bureau.

Hill, M., Laybourn, A. and Borland, M. (1996) 'Engaging with primary aged children about their emotions and well-being: methodological considerations', *Children and Society* 10: 129–144.

Hill, M. and Shaw, M. (1998) *Signposts in Adoption: Policy, Practice and Research Issues*, London: British Agencies for Adoption and Fostering.

Home Office (1959) *Appendix to Home Office Letter, HO* 58/59, March, 1959.

Hoopes, J. L., Shermane, E. A., Lawder, E. A., Andrews, R. G. and Lower, K. D. (1970) *A Follow Up Study of Adoptions: Post-Placement Functioning of Adopted Children*, New York: Child Welfare League of America.

Hopkinson Committee, (1921) *Report of the Committee on Child Adoption*, Cmd 1254, London: HMSO.

Horsburgh Committee (1937) *Report of the Departmental Committee on Adoption Societies and Agencies*, Cmd 5499, London: HMSO.

Houghton Committee (1970) *Working Paper Containing the Provisional Proposals of the Departmental Committee on the Adoption of Children*, London: HMSO.

Houghton Committee (1972) *Report of the Departmental Committee on the Adoption of Children*, Cmnd 5107, London: HMSO.

Howe, D. (1996) *Adopters on Adoption: Reflection on Parenthood and Children*, London: British Agencies for Adoption and Fostering.

Howe, D. and Feast, J. (2000) *Adoption, Search and Reunion: the Long-term Experience of Adopted Adults*, London: The Children's Society.

Howe, D., Sawbridge, P. and Hinings, D. (1992) *Half a Million Women: Mothers Who Lose Their Children by Adoption*, London: Penguin.

Hughes, B. (1995) 'Openness and contact in adoption: a child-centred perspective', *British Journal of Social Work* 25, 6: 729–747.

Hughes, B. and Logan, J. (1993) *The Hidden Dimension*, London: Mental Health Foundation.

Hurst Committee (1954) *Report of the Departmental Committee on the Adoption of Children*, Cmd 9248, London: HMSO.

Hussell, C. and Monaghan, B. (1982) 'Going for good', *Social Work To-day* 13, 47: 7–9.

Interdepartmental Working Group (1992) *Review of Adoption Law: a Consultation Document*, London: Department of Health and Welsh Office.

Ivaldi, G. (1998) *Children Adopted from Care: Examination of Agency Adoptions in England–1996*, London: British Agencies for Adoption and Fostering.

Ivaldi, G. (2000) *Surveying Adoption: a Comprehensive Analysis of Local Authority Adoptions 1998–1999 (England)*, London: British Agencies for Adoption and Fostering.

Iwanek, M. (1987) *A Study of Open Adoption Placements*, New Zealand: Petone.

Jaffee, B. and Fanshel, D. (1970) *How They Fared in Adoption: a Follow Up Study*, New York: Columbia University Press.

James, A, and Prout, A. (eds) (1997) *Constructing and Reconstructing Childhood: Contemporary Issues in the Sociological Study of Childhood*, 2nd edn, London: Falmer.

John, M. (1996) *Children in Charge: the Child's Right to a Fair Hearing*, London: Jessica Kingsley.

Jones, M. (2002) 'Orders or agreements?' in H. Argent (ed.) *Staying Connected: Managing Contact Arrangements in Adoption*, London: British Agencies for Adoption and Fostering.

Kadushin, A. (1970) *Adopting Older Children*, New York: Columbia University Press.

Kedward, C., Luckward, B. and Lawson, H. (1999) 'Mediation and post-adoption contact: the early experience of the post-adoption centre contact mediation service', *Adoption and Fostering* 23, 3: 16–26.

Kellmer Pringle, M. L. (1967) *Adoption – Facts and Fallacies*, London: Longmans.

King, P. (1994) 'The role of the guardian *ad litem* in contested adoptions' in M. Ryburn (ed.) *Contested Adoptions: Research, Law Policy and Practice*, Aldershot: Arena.

Kirk, D. (1964) *Shared Fate*, London: Collier Macmillan.

Kornitzer, M. (1968) *Adoption and Family Life*, London: Putnam.

Kosonen, M. (1996) 'Maintaining sibling relationships: a neglected dimension in child-care practice', *British Journal of Social Work*, 26: 809–822.

Krugman, D. C. (1964) 'Reality in adoption', *Child Welfare* 43: 349–358.

Lacey-Smith, C. and Aldgate, J. (1992) *Open Adoption: a Survey of Adoptive Parents and Their Children*, Oxford: Oxford Diocesan Council for Social Work.

Lamb, M. E. and Sutton-Smith, B. (eds) (1982) *Sibling Relationships: Their Nature and Significance across the Lifespan*, London: Lawrence Erlbaum Associates.

Lansdown, G. (1994) 'The welfare of the child in contested proceedings' in M. Ryburn (ed.) *Contested Adoptions: Research, Law Policy and Practice*, Aldershot: Arena.

Law Commission of New Zealand (2000) *Adoption and Its Alternatives: a Different Approach and New Framework*, Report 65, Wellington, New Zealand: Law Commission.

Lawton, J. and Gross, S. Z. (1964) 'Review of psychiatric literature on adopted children', *Archives of General Psychiatry* 11: 635–644.

Lewis, A. and Lindsay, G. (eds) (2000) *Researching Children's Perspectives*, Buckingham: Open University Press.

Lindley, B. (1997) 'Open adoption is the door a-jar?', *Child and Family Law Quarterly* 9, 2: 115–129.

Lockridge, F. (1947) *Adopting a Child*, New York: Greenberg.

Logan, J. (1996) 'Birth mothers and their mental health: uncharted territory', *British Journal of Social Work* 26: 609–625.

Logan, J. (1999) 'Exchanging information post-adoption: the views of adoptive parents and birth parents', *Adoption and Fostering* 23, 3: 27–38.

Lord, J. and Borthwick, S. (2001) *Together or Apart? Assessing Brothers and Sisters for Permanent Placement*, London: British Agencies for Adoption and Fostering.

Lowe, N. (1997) 'The changing face of adoption – the gift/donation model versus the contract/services model', *Child and Family Law Quarterly* 9, 4: 371–386.

Lowe, N., Murch, M., Borkowski, M., Weaver, A., Beckford, V. and Thomas, C. (1999) *Supporting Adoption: Reframing the Approach*, London: British Agencies for Adoption and Fostering.

Macaskill, C. (1985) *Against the Odds: Adopting Mentally Handicapped Children*, London: British Agencies for Adoption and Fostering.

Macaskill, C. (2002) *Safe Contact: Children in Permanent Placement and Contact with Their Birth Relatives*, Lyme Regis: Russell House Publishing.

Mason, K. and Selman, P. (1997) 'Birth parents' experiences of contested adoption', *Adoption and Fostering* 21, 1: 21–28.

Mason, K. and Selman, P. (1998) 'British parents' experience of contested adoption' in M. Hill and M. Shaw (eds) *Signposts in Adoption: Policy, Practice and Research Issues*, London: British Agencies for Adoption and Fostering.

Masson, J. (2000a) 'Thinking about contact – a social or legal problem?', *Child and Family Law Quarterly* 12, 1: 15–29.

Masson, J. (2000b) 'Researching children's perspectives: legal issues' in A. Lewis and G. Lindsay (eds) *Researching Children's Perspectives*, Buckingham: Open University Press.

Masson, J., Harrison, C. and Pavlovic, A. (1999) *Working with Children and Lost Parents: Putting Partnership into Practice*, York: York Publishing Services.

Mayall, B. (ed.) (1994) *Children's Childhoods: Observed and Experienced*, London: Falmer Press.

McKay, M. (1980) 'Planning for permanent placement', *Adoption and Fostering* 99: 19–21.

McRoy, R. G. (1991) 'American experience and research on openness', *Adoption and Fostering* 15, 4: 99–111.

McWhinnie, A. (1967) *Adopted Children: How They Group Up*, London: Routledge and Kegan Paul.

McWhinnie, A. (1994) 'The concept of open adoption – how valid is it?' in A. McWhinnie and J. Smith (eds) *Current Human Dilemmas in Adoption*, Dundee: University of Dundee.

Morris, C. (1984) *The Permanency Principle in Child Care Social Work*, Norwich: University of East Anglia.

Morrow, V. (1998) *Understanding Families: Children's Perspectives*, London: National Children's Bureau.

Morrow, V. and Richards, M. (1996) 'The ethics of social research with children: an overview', *Children and Society*, 10: 99–105.

Mullender, A. (1991) *Open Adoption: the Philosophy and the Practice*, London: British Agencies for Adoption and Fostering.

Mullender, A. (1999) *We are Family: Sibling Relationships in Placement and Beyond*, London: British Agencies for Adoption and Fostering.

Murch, M., Lowe, N., Borkowski, M., Copner, R. and Griew, K. (1993) *Pathways to Adoption*, London: HMSO.

Neil, E. (1999) 'The sibling relationships of adopted children and patterns of contact after adoption' in A. Mullender (ed.) *We Are Family: Sibling Relationships in Placement and Beyond*, London: British Agencies for Adoption and Fostering.

Neil, E. (2000) 'The reasons why young children are placed for adoption: findings from a recently placed sample and implications for future identity issues', *Child and Family Social Work* 5, 4: 303–316.

Neil, E. (2002a) 'Contact after adoption: the role of agencies in making and supporting plans', *Adoption and Fostering* 26, 1: 25–38.

Neil, E. (2002b) 'Managing face-to-face contact for young adopted children' in H. Argent (ed.) *Staying Connected: Managing Contact Arrangements in Adoption*, London: British Agencies for Adoption and Fostering.

Nelson, K. (1985) *On the Frontier of Adoption: a Study of Special Needs Adopted Children*, New York: Child Welfare League Of America.

Owen, M. (1999) 'Single adopters and sibling groups' in A. Mullender (ed.) *We Are Family: Sibling Relationships in Placement and Beyond*, London: British Agencies for Adoption and Fostering.

Pacheco, F. and Eme, R. (1993) 'An outcome study of the reunion between adoptees and biological parents', *Child Welfare* 72: 53–64.

Parker, R. (1971) *Planning for Deprived Children*, London: National Children's Homes.

Parker, R. (1999) *Adoption Now: Messages from Research*, Chichester: John Wiley And Sons.

Parton, N. (1991) *Governing the Family*, London: Macmillan.

Parton, N. (1996a) 'The new politics of child protection' in J. Pilcher and S. Wragg (eds) *Thatcher's Children*, London: Falmer Press.

Parton, N. (1996b) 'Social work, risk and the blaming system' in N. Parton (ed.) *Social Theory, Social Change and Social Work*, London: Routledge.

Parton, N. (ed.) (1997) *Child Protection and Family Support: Tensions, Contradictions and Possibilities*, London: Routledge.

Parton, N. (1998) 'Risk, advanced liberalism and child welfare: the need to rediscover uncertainty and ambiguity', *British Journal of Social Work* 28, 1: 5–28.

Peller, L. (1961) 'About telling the child of his adoption', *Bulletin of the Philadelphia Association for Psychoanalysis*, 11: 145–154.

Performance and Innovation Unit (2000) *The Prime Minister's Review of Adoption*, London: Performance and Innovation Unit.

Pitcher, D. (2002) 'Placement with grandparents: the issues for grandparents who care for their grandchildren', *Adoption and Fostering* 26, 1: 6–14.

Quinton, D., Rushton, A., Dance, C. and Mayes, D. (1997) 'Contact between children placed away from home and their birth parents: research issues and evidence', *Clinical Child Psychology and Psychiatry* 2, 3: 393–413.

Quinton, D., Selwyn, J., Rushton, A. and Dance, C. (1998) 'Contact with birth parents in adoption – a response to Ryburn', *Child and Family Law Quarterly* 10, 4: 1–14.

Quinton, D., Selwyn, J., Rushton, A. and Dance, C. (1999) 'Contact with children placed away from home and their birth parents: Ryburn's reanalysis analysed', *Clinical Child Psychology and Psychiatry* 4, 4: 519–531.

Qvortrup, J. (1987) 'Introduction', *International Journal of Sociology* 17, 3: 3–37.

Reddy, S. G. (1996) 'Claims to expert knowledge and the subversion of democracy: the triumph of risk over uncertainty', *Economy and Society* 25: 222–54.

Reeves, S. and Dolan, P. (1978) 'A Retrospective Assessment of Adoption', *Clearing House for Local Authority Social Services Research* 8: 83–126.

Registrar General (2001) *Marriage, Divorce and Adoption Statistics*, London: Office for National Statistics.

Reitz, M. and Watson, K. W. (1992) *Adoption and the Family System*, New York: Guilford.

Robinson, E. (2000) *Adoption and Loss – the Hidden Grief*, Christies Beach, Southern Australia: Clova Publications.

Robinson, E. (2002) 'Post-adoption grief counselling', *Adoption and Fostering* 26, 2: 57–63.

Roche, H. and Perlesz, A. (2000) 'A legitimate choice and voice: the experience of adult adopters who have chosen not to search for their biological families', *Adoption and Fostering* 24, 2: 8–19.

Rockel, J. and Ryburn, M. (1988) *Adoption Today: Change and Choice in New Zealand*, Auckland, New Zealand: Heinemann Reed.

Roll, J. (2001) *The Adoption and Children Bill, House of Commons Research Paper 01/33*, London: House of Commons Library.

Rowe, J. (1966) *Parents, Children and Adoption*, London: Routledge and Kegan Paul.

Rowe, J. and Lambert, L. (1973) *Children Who Wait*, London: Association of British Adoption Agencies.

Rushton, A., Dance, C., Quinton, D. and Mayes, D. (2001) *Siblings in Late Permanent Placements*, London: British Agencies for Adoption and Fostering.

Ryan, M. (1994) 'Contested proceedings: justice and the law' in M. Ryburn (ed.) *Contested Adoptions: Research, Law Policy and Practice*, Aldershot: Arena.

Ryburn, M. (1992) *Adoption in the 1990's: Identity and Openness*, Royal Leamington Spa: Leamington Press.

Ryburn, M. (1994) 'The use of an adversarial process in contested adoptions' in M. Ryburn (ed.) *Contested Adoptions: Research, Law, Policy and Practice*, Aldershot: Arena.

Ryburn, M. (1995) 'Adopted children's identity and information needs', *Children and Society* 9, 3: 41–64.

Ryburn, M. (1996) 'A study of post-adoption contact in compulsory adoptions', *British Journal of Social Work* 26, 5: 627–646.

Ryburn, M. (1997a) 'Welfare and justice in post-adoption contact', *Family Law* 27: 28–37.

Ryburn, M. (1997b) 'The uneven scales of justice: private law contact applications in divorce and adoption', *Adoption and Fostering* 21, 3: 23–34.

Ryburn, M. (1998) 'In whose best interests? – post adoption contact with the birth family', *Child and Family Law Quarterly* 10, 1: 53–70.

Ryburn, M. (1999) 'Contact between children and their birth parents: a reanalysis of the evidence in relation to permanent placements', *Clinical Child Psychology and Psychiatry* 4, 4: 505–518.

Sachdev, P. (1991) 'Achieving openness in adoption: some critical issues in policy formation', *American Journal of Orthopsychiatry* 61, 2: 241–249.

Sants, H. J. (1964) 'Genealogical bewilderment in children with substitute parents', *British Journal of Medical Psychology* 37: 133–141.

Savas, D. and Treece, S. (1998) 'Adoption or residence? too many parents . . .?', *Child and Family Law Quarterly* 10, 3: 31–320.

Save the Children (2000) *Children's Rights: Equal Rights? Diversity, Difference and the Issue of Discrimination*, London: the International Save the Children Alliance.

Sawbridge, P. (1983) *Parents for Children*, London: British Agencies for Adoption and Fostering.

Schaffer, H. (1990) *Making Decisions about Children*, Oxford: Blackwell.

Schechter, M. D. and Bertocci, D. (1990) 'The meaning of the search' in D. Brodzinsky and M. Schechter (eds) *The Psychology of Adoption*, New York: Oxford University Press

Schwartz, E. M. (1970) 'The family romance fantasy in children adopted in infancy', *Child Welfare* XLIX, 7: 386–391.

Scottish Office (1993) *The Future of Adoption Law in Scotland: a Consultation Paper*, Edinburgh: Scottish Office.

Scottish Office (1997) *Scotland's Children: The Children (Scotland) Act 1995, Regulations and Guidance, Volume 2*, Edinburgh: The Stationery Office.

Secretary of State for Health (1993) *Adoption: the Future*, Cm 2288 London: HMSO.

Secretary of State for Health (1998) *Modernising Social Services: Promoting Independence, Improving Protection and Raising Standards*, CM4169, London: Department of Health.

Secretary of State for Health (2000) *Adoption: a New Approach*, CM 5017, London: Department of Health.

Seglow, J., Kellmer Pringle, E. and Wedge, P. (1972) *Growing Up Adopted*, Windsor: National Foundation for Educational Research in England and Wales.

Siegel, D. H. (1993) 'Open adoption of infants: adoptive parents' perceptions of advantages and disadvantages', *Social Work* 38, 1: 15–23.

Silverstein, D. and Kaplan Roszia, S. (1999) 'Openness: a critical component of special needs adoption', *Child Welfare* 78, 5: 637–651.

Smith, C. (1997) 'Children's rights: judicial ambivalence and social resistance', *International Journal of Law, Policy and the Family* 11: 103–139.

Smith, C. and Logan, J. (2002) 'Adoptive parenthood as a "legal fiction" – its consequences for direct post-adoption contact', *Child and Family Law Quarterly* 14, 3: 281–301.

Sorosky, A. D., Baran, A. and Pannor, R. (1975) 'Identity conflicts in adoption', *American Journal of Orthopsychiatry*, 45, 1: 18–27.

Stancombe, J. and White, S. (1998) 'Psychotherapy without foundations? Hermeneutics, discourse and the end of certainty', *Theory and Psychology* 8, 5: 579–599.

Stevenson, P. S. (1976) 'The evaluation of adoption reunions in British Columbia', *Social Work* 4: 9–12.

Striker, S. and Kimmel, E. (1979) *The Anti-Colouring Book*, London: Scholastic Publications.

Swindells, H., Neves, A., Kushner, M. and Skilbeck, R. (1999) *Family Law and the Human Rights Act 1998*, Bristol: Jordan Publishing Limited.

Sykes, M. (2000) 'Adoption with contact: a study of adoptive parents and the impact of continuing contact with the family of origin', *Adoption and Fostering* 24, 2: 20–32.

Thoburn, J. (1990) *Interdepartmental Review of Adoption Law Background Paper Number 2: Review of Research Relating to Adoption*, London: Department of Health.

Thoburn, J., Norford, L. and Parvez Rashid, S. (2000) *Permanent Family Placement for Children of Minority Ethnic Origin*, London: Jessica Kingsley.

Thomas, C., Beckford, V., Lowe, N. and Murch, M. (1999) *Adopted Children Speaking*, London: British Agencies for Adoption and Fostering.

Thomas, N. and O'Kane, C. (1998a) 'The ethics of participatory research with children', *Children and Society* 12: 336–348.

Thomas, N. and O' Kane, C. (1998b) *Children and Decision Making: a Summary Report*, University of Wales, Swansea: International Centre for Childhood Studies.

Tizard, B. (1977) *Adoption – a Second Chance*, London: Open Books.

Tomlin (1925) *Child Adoption Committee: First Report*, Cmd. 2401, London: HMSO.

Tomlin (1926a) *Child Adoption Committee: Second Report*, Cmd 2469, London: HMSO.

Tomlin (1926b) *Child Adoption Committee: Third Report*, Cmd 2711, London: HMSO.

Triseliotis, J. (1970) *Evaluation of Social Policy and Practice*, Edinburgh: Edinburgh University.

Triseliotis, J. (1973) *In Search of Origins*, London: Routledge and Kegan Paul.

Triseliotis, J. (1983) 'Identity and security in long-term fostering and adoption', *Adoption and Fostering* 7: 22–31.

Triseliotis, J. (1985) 'Adoption with contact', *Adoption and Fostering* 9, 4: 19–24.

Triseliotis, J. (1991) 'Open adoption' in A. Mullender (ed.) *Open Adoption: the Philosophy and the Practice*, London: British Agencies for Adoption and Fostering.

Triseliotis, J. (1993) 'Open adoption – The evidence examined' in M. Adcock, J. Kaniuk and R. White (eds) *Exploring Openness in Adoption*, Croydon: Significant Publications.

Triseliotis, J. (2002) 'Long term foster care or adoption? The evidence examined', *Child and Family Social Work* 7, 1: 23–35.

Triseliotis, J. and Hill, M. (1990) 'Contrasting adoption, foster and residential care' in D. M. Brodzinsky and M. D. Schechter (eds) *The Psychology of Adoption*, New York: Oxford University Press.

Triseliotis, J., Shireman, J. and Hundleby, M. (1997) *Adoption: Theory, Policy and Practice*, London: Cassell.

Utting, Sir William (1991) *Children in the Public Care – a Review of Residential Care*, London: Department of Health.

Utting, Sir William (1997) *People Like Us: the Report of the Review of the Safeguards for Children Living Away From Home*, London: Department of Health.

Van Bueren, G. (1995) 'Children's access to adoption records – state discretion or an enforceable international right?', *Modern Law Review* 58, 1: 37–53.

Waterhouse, Sir Ronald (2000) *The Report of the Tribunal of Enquiry into the Abuse of Children in Care in the Former County Council Areas of Gwynedd and Clwyd Since 1974*, London: The Stationery Office.

Wedge, P. and Mantle, G. (1991) *Sibling Groups in Social Work: a Study of Children Referred for Permanent Substitute Family Placements*, Aldershot: Avebury.

Wells, S. (1993) 'Post traumatic stress disorder in birth mothers', *Adoption and Fostering* 17, 2: 30–32.

Whitaker, D., Cook, J., Dunne, C. and Rocliffe, S. (1984) *The Experience of Residential Care from the Perspectives of Children, Parents and Care-Givers*, University of York: Department of Social Policy and Social Work.

White, S. (1997) 'Beyond retroduction? Hermeneutics, reflexivity and social work practice', *British Journal of Social Work* 27: 739–54.

Wieder, H. (1977) 'The family romance fantasies of adopted children', *Psycho-Analytical Quarterly* 46, 2: 155–200.

Winkler, R. C. and Van Keppel, M. (1984) *Relinquishing Mothers in Adoption: Their Long-Term Adjustment*, Monograph Number 3, Melbourne: Institute of Family Studies.

Witmer, H. L., Herzog, E., Weinstein, E. A. and Sullivan, M. E. (1963) *Independent Adoptions: a Follow Up Study*, New York: Russell Sage Foundation.

Young, J. (1999) *The Exclusive Society*, London: Sage.

# Index

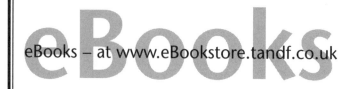